the NATURAL BEAUTY SOLUTION

Break Free from Commercial Beauty Products
Using Simple Recipes and Natural Ingredients

MARY HELEN LEONARD

PHOTOGRAPHY BY
KIMBERLY DAVIS

SPRING HOUSE PRESS

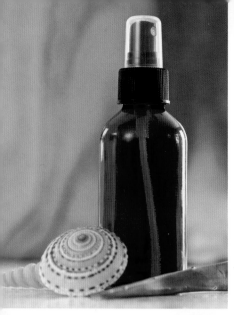
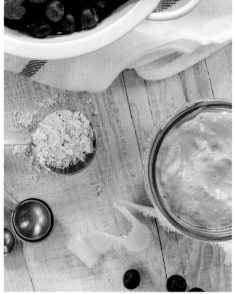
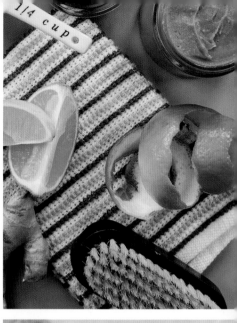
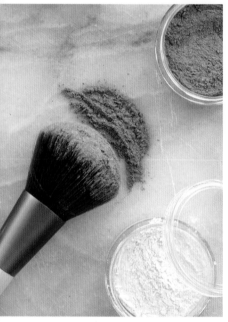
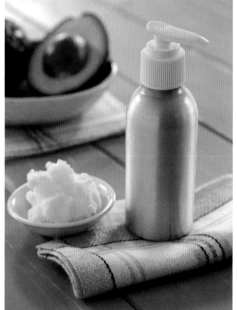
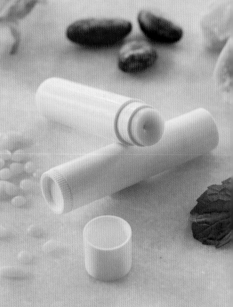

Publisher: Paul McGahren
Editor: Matthew Teague
Designer: Lindsay Hess
Photographer: Kimberly Davis
Copyeditor: Teresa Dulaney Dewald
Indexer: Holly Day

Spring House Press
3613 Brush Hill Court
Nashville, TN 37216

ISBN: 978-1-940611-18-1

Library of Congress Control Number: 2015932165

Printed in China

First Printing: June 2015

The information in this book is presented in good faith; however, no warranty is given, nor are results guaranteed. Your safety is your responsibility. Neither Spring House Press nor the author assumes any responsibility for any injuries or accidents.

The following manufacturers/names appearing in *The Natural Beauty Solution* are trademarks: Environmental Working Group, Jolly Rancher, Blythe Natural Living, Vermont Soap, Austin Natural Soap, Bramble Berry, FDA, INCI, USDA National Organic Program, Artifact Girl, Chapstick

To learn more about Spring House Press books, or to find a retailer near you, email *info@springhousepress.com* or visit us at *www.springhousepress.com*.

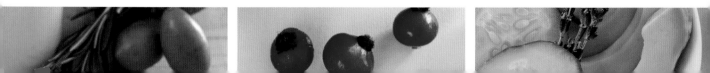

Acknowledgments

I've always been an overconfident person. I was the type of kid who would launch herself from boulders or out of windows, surviving such leaps only by the special grace that preserves fools and little children. While maturity has granted me with a deeper respect for my physical well-being, that spirit of reckless ambition is still very much a part of who I am.

So when the stars aligned to grant me my first baby and my first book deal simultaneously, I graciously accepted the challenge. I had just eight months to write my manuscript, and my baby was due smack-dab in the middle of it. It turns out I had seriously underestimated how hard it would be to write a book or to care for an infant, nevermind doing both while holding down a full-time job.

Lucky for me, that special grace is no longer the only thing that preserves me. While working on this book I was blessed with boundless support from my family, friends, and colleagues. My mother spent countless hours bouncing my son on her knee, helping me with laundry, and making sure I stayed fed. When I say this book could not have been written without her help I mean it very literally.

My husband was there to cheer me on, even when I doubted the possibility of making it through this project with my sanity intact. He believed I could do it, as he seems to believe I can do anything. His faith in me is the best gift a girl could ask for.

My sister, Heather, has read this book more times than anyone (except maybe me) supplying edits, questions, and a second point of view every step of the way. I was so lucky to have her on my side, offering me her advice and support.

I'd like to thank Sally Ekus, my agent, for taking an interest in this project and also in me. I knew I wanted to write this book one day, but it took meeting Sally for me to realize that waiting for "one day" wasn't a great plan. Sally gave me the tools I needed to turn a daydream into a goal, and from a goal into a book.

I feel very lucky to have worked with Paul McGahren, Matthew Teague, Lindsay Hess, and Kimberly Davis on this book. From the very start I could tell that we shared a vision for how it would all come together. This is my first book, but I imagine it is a rare thing to have the author, publisher, editor, designer, and photographer work together so effortlessly. I'm grateful for the talents, wisdom, and creativity of these people who turned my words into paper and pictures.

Thanks to my amazing friends, fellow bloggers, tweeters, and DIY geniuses. I'm grateful to be part of such a supportive community both locally in Austin and online. And thanks to Nelly for modeling and for letting us shoot photos in her gorgeous kitchen!

Finally, my thanks go out to Jay Basu and Kibby Mitra. I had no idea where my job at From Nature With Love would take me when I showed up in a blizzard for my interview back in 2005. They gave me the opportunity to learn and create for a living, and I've done my best to make the most of it over the years. My head is fit to burst with the knowledge I've gained while writing *The Natural Beauty Workshop* blog, and I'm glad to be able to share what I've learned through this book. Jay and Kibby have been incredibly supportive of this project, both as professionals and as friends.

They say that many hands make light work. I'm eternally grateful for every hand involved in the making of this book. Here's to many more.

CONTENTS

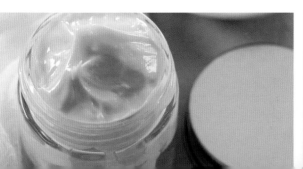
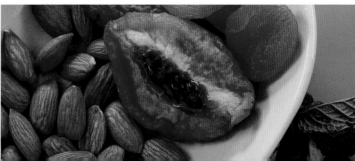

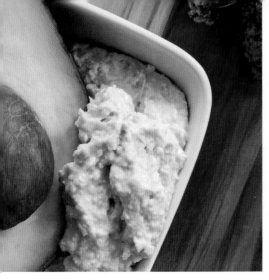
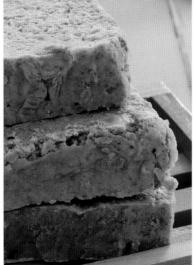

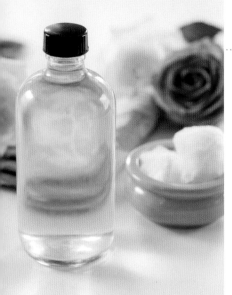
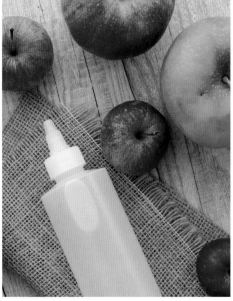
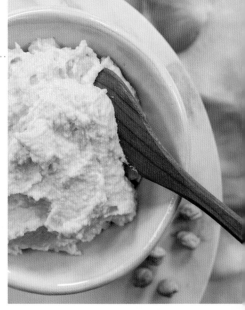
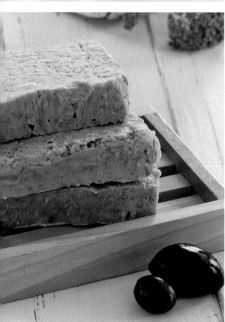
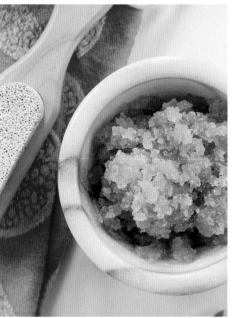
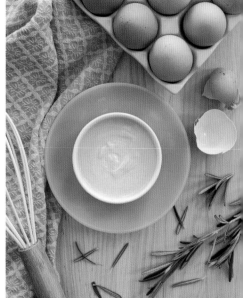
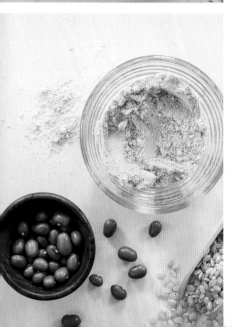
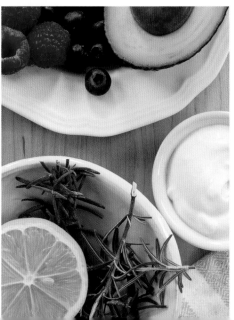
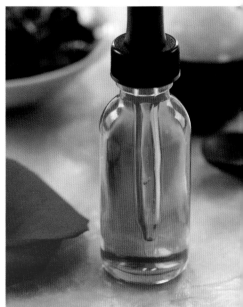

Why Go Natural?

A SIMPLE STEP TOWARD HEALTHIER LIVING

Your refrigerator is packed with fresh veggies. You have organic grains in the pantry and have made a concerted effort to cut down on things like fast food and processed snacks. You are well on your way to a healthier lifestyle. But have you taken a look in your bathroom lately? Commercial skincare products are produced with some pretty nasty ingredients. Chemical preservatives, synthetic fragrances, questionable additives, and controversial ingredients are found in just about every bottle on the shelf.

We cover ourselves in this stuff from head to toe—often spending quite a bit of money to do so—all for the promise of clear skin and lustrous hair. Yet many times the very products that promise to deliver these things are causing irritation, damage, and possibly even illness. Watchdog organizations such as The Environmental Working Group (*www.ewg.org*) do their best to keep track of harmful ingredients and fight to have them removed from beauty products, but for every ingredient that is banned another crops up to take its place.

Navigating the world of commercial beauty in search of products that are both safe and effective can be expensive and daunting. Creating your own simple products at home is a surprisingly easy and affordable solution to this issue. Not only will making your own products help you avoid dangerous ingredients—it can help get your skin and hair on the way to looking and feeling better naturally.

This book is meant to be your companion as you make the leap into a new beauty routine that uses natural ingredients to bring out your body's inherent ability for self-care. When you break free from the cycle of over-drying and skin-clogging that commercial beauty products create, our bodies have a way of regulating themselves. For example, our scalps stop over-producing sebum (our skin's natural conditioning oil) just days after shampooing is stopped. Over the next few weeks sebum production starts and stops as our body figures out just how much is needed to protect and condition the hair. Within a year, the scalp settles in to a natural rhythm that eliminates the need for additional conditioners or hair oils altogether.

Our bodies know what to do to keep our skin and hair healthy. This book isn't about adding extra potions and promises to an already-full world of beauty products. It's about simplifying what you put on your body, encouraging your skin and hair to care for itself, and helping to keep it on track while it does so.

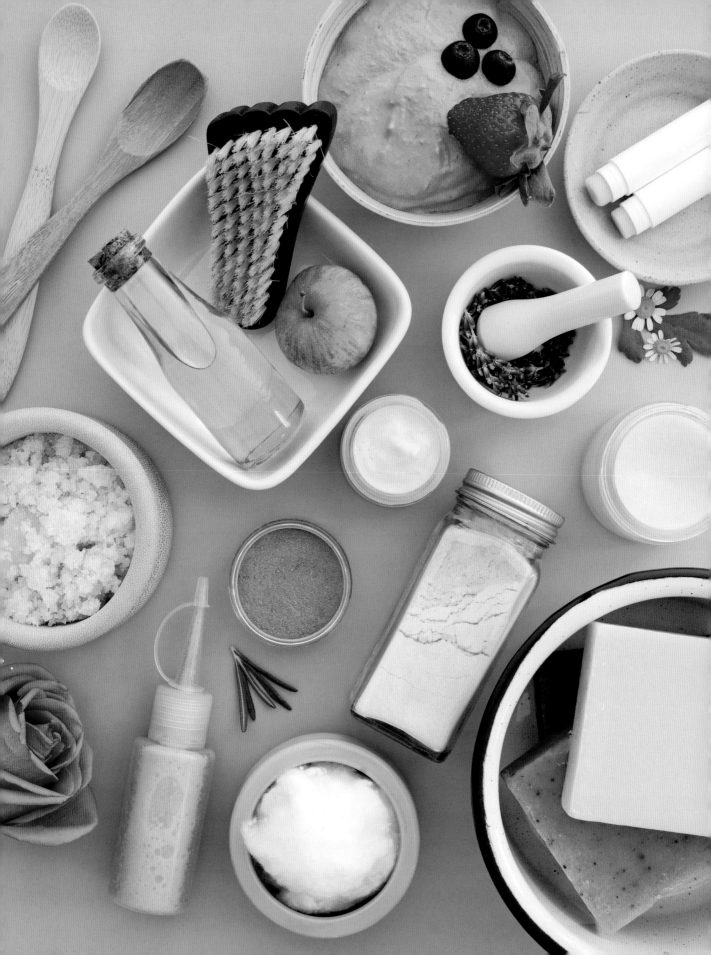

GETTING STARTED

While you are more than welcome to browse through this book and pick out recipes as you please, it is my hope that you will feel inspired to embrace natural beauty for your entire routine. Just like switching to a healthier diet or beginning an exercise routine, making the leap to natural beauty really is a lifestyle change. In either case, I recommend taking it slow by replacing one product at a time or focusing on one aspect of your routine at a time.

The everyday recipes in this book are given in the simplest form possible. You will find options to customize them to suit your particular needs. It's always a good idea to start off with the basic version of each recipe. Once you see how your skin and hair react to that simple version, you can add or replace ingredients to better suit your needs. »

Most of the ingredients used in the basic versions of the everyday recipes are listed in Chapter 2: Building Your Pantry. These ingredients are used most often in a standard natural beauty routine. Browse the ingredients to learn about how they work, where you can find them, and how they should be used.

I've also included specialty recipes in this book that go beyond the essential parts of your routine. These recipes use less common ingredients than are found in Chapter 2, and make a great introduction into more advanced skin care formulation. Specialty recipes for things like facial masques or pedicure treatments are sort of like icing on the natural beauty cake. They aren't strictly necessary, but they can be fun. I recommend exploring them after you get your everyday routine worked out.

TOXIC BEAUTY INGREDIENTS

Parabens

Commercial products are formulated to last a very long time. Think about how long products might sit on the store shelf and then how long they are kept in your bathroom cabinet. It takes heavy-duty preservatives to prevent products from becoming overrun with bacteria, mold, and other nasty microbes. *Parabens* are preservatives commonly used in skin and hair care products. But they have a dark side: According to certain studies, parabens may cause health issues such as endocrine disruption, reproductive toxicity, and immune system toxicity—a high price to pay for shelf-stable products!

YOUR FIRST STEPS

As with any lifestyle change, you may find it easier to give yourself a head start. I suggest kicking things off with a bathroom cabinet cleanse. This gives you the chance to scrutinize your existing routine. Next you can develop a plan for replacing your products with new, customized recipes.

STEP ONE: CABINET CLEANSE

Start by taking out all of your skin care, hair care, and body care products. Line them up, grouped by their purpose. For example, you might have one group of hair care products, another for facial care, and another for bath and body.

Go through the products one by one, discarding any that are very old or expired. Consider the products that are left. How often do you use them? How much do you like them? Set aside the products that you use most often, and the ones that you enjoy using the most. Make a list of these products so that you'll know what needs to be replaced. You can use the form provided on page 126 of the Appendix to keep track of the products you'd like to replace. As for the rest, consider passing them on to friends or family before tossing them out.

Seek out natural and handmade replacements for products on your list from the resources listed on page 122. Be sure to note how you plan to replace each product. Then use this information to make a shopping list of ingredients you'll need.

STEP TWO: REPLACE YOUR COMMERCIAL PRODUCTS

A great way to start your natural routine is to continue to use your favorite products until they run out! When you notice your favorite store-bought product running low, gather the ingredients you need to create its homemade replacement. By replacing products one by one you can minimize the expense of starting a new routine and make the process easier. Taking things slowly also gives your body time to adjust to the new products and techniques one at a time, which helps you identify any issues you might run into along the way.

Keep swapping out products as your commercial items run out. Before you know it, your entire routine will be revamped! If you run into any products that are particularly tough along the way, try reaching out to others in the natural beauty community. You'll find a list of blogs, forums, and informational sites in the Resources section.

TOXIC BEAUTY INGREDIENTS

Phthalates

Phthalates (pronounced "thal-ates") are a little harder to spot than other toxic beauty ingredients. This is because they are usually found within a fragrance and aren't listed separately. It takes extra legwork to find out whether or not a store-bought product contains phthalates. Why should you bother to keep an eye out for phthalates? Like parabens, phthalates have possible connections to reproductive toxicity and endocrine disruption. They are also linked to developmental issues, making their safety questionable for pregnant women, nursing moms, kids, babies, and pretty much everyone else.

STEP THREE: CUSTOMIZE YOUR RECIPES

As you replace products from your routine you'll start to notice what does and doesn't work for you. Is your skin dry? Is your hair heavier or more oily than you'd like? Many of the everyday recipes in this book contain information on customization and troubleshooting. Once your routine is established, it's a good idea to take a close look at each segment and make any necessary adjustments.

If you have a condition such as eczema, psoriasis, or chronic dry skin, pay extra attention to how your skin reacts to new recipes, ingredients, or changes to your routine. If you are under a doctor or dermatologist's care, discuss your natural beauty plan with them before you get started.

INGREDIENTS: WATER, SODIUM LAURYL SULFATE, SODIUM LAURETH SULFATE, COCAMIDOPROPYL BETAINE, SODIUM CHLORIDE, GLYCOL DISTEARATE, CITRIC ACID, SODIUM CITRATE, SODIUM XYLENESULFONATE, FRAGRANCE, DIMETHICONE, SODIUM BENZOATE, POLYQUATERNIUM-76, TETRASODIUM EDTA, NO. PANTHENYL ETHYL ETHER, METHYLCHLOROISOTHIAZOLINONE, METHYLISOTHIAZOLINONE.

MADE IN U.S.A. of U.S. and/or Imported ingredients

The next time you pick up a bottle of shower gel, take a look at the ingredient list. You may be surprised how many ingredients go into something as simple as liquid soap.

KEEP IT SIMPLE

If you do a little searching, you can dig up plenty of recipe books for natural beauty. The biggest difference between this book and many other natural beauty books is that the recipes in this book are given in their most simplified form. While experimenting with exotic ingredients and complex formulas can be fun, keeping things simple is the best strategy for establishing an everyday routine. Everyday skin care and hair care is similar to everyday cooking and eating. The healthiest options often depend on simple combinations of high quality ingredients. Quality over quantity matters. For example, a great facial oil doesn't have to contain twenty different ingredients: Just one or two that work really well will suffice.

FRESH IS BEST

Commercial beauty products have been formulated by scientists to remain shelf stable. Mass-produced recipes won't go bad before their expiration date and are built to withstand direct handling and less than ideal storage. Handmade products don't have the protection of high-powered preservatives so keeping them fresh depends on proper storing and handling.

We aren't used to thinking of beauty products in the same way that we do food but, the truth is, they are often made from very similar stuff. You wouldn't want to eat a meal that has been left on the kitchen counter overnight, and a fresh batch of handmade lotion is very much the same.

The best way to safely use homemade products is to make them to order. Create products in small batches, use them up quickly, and always try to handle products and ingredients with clean hands.

DEVELOP A ROUTINE

Sometimes you have to kiss a few frogs before you find your Prince Charming. Falling in love with your natural beauty routine could take a little bit of trial and error as well. Not every recipe or technique will work for you right away. Sometimes it takes a little tweaking and a lot of practice to get something to work for you. Other times, you may find that you need a different method altogether. As you try different recipes and new ingredients, take note of how your skin and hair react. By continuing to make adjustments along the way you'll end up creating a routine that is fully customized to your unique needs.

TOXIC BEAUTY INGREDIENTS

Sulfates

If you look at the label on store-bought shampoo, body wash or bar soap, you are likely to see an ingredient containing the word *sulfate*. Sulfates are types of detergents and surfactants that help create that rich, bubbly lather that we all love. Unfortunately, they also have a habit of stripping the skin of the beneficial oils that keep it moisturized and protected. People with sensitive skin sometimes have very strong reactions to sulfates. Reactions can result in redness, rashes, and, in extreme cases, bleeding. Sodium Laureth Sulfate (also referred to as SLS) is one of the most common sulfates found in bath and body products, and is one of many sulfate ingredients that can wreak havoc on your skin and scalp.

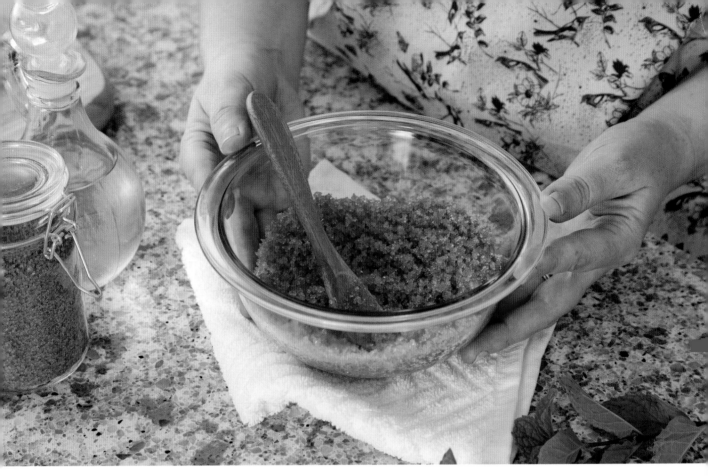

Most natural beauty recipes are very easy to make. The sugar scrub above can be made by mixing just two ingredients—sugar and oil.

In order to establish a natural beauty routine that really works you need to do four things:

Give each recipe, ingredient, or method a fair shot. Your skin needs time to adjust any time you change a routine. It's important to let that adjustment happen before you decide whether or not something works for you. As a general rule, it's good to give any change about seven days to settle in. There are a few exceptions that I'll mention along the way. However, if your skin or hair has an extreme reaction or if you suspect you might be having an allergic reaction to an ingredient, stop using it right away and consult your doctor.

Pay attention to your body. Your skin and hair have a way of telling you what they need. Paying close attention to how your body reacts to the recipes you use can help clue you in to how they can be adjusted to better suit your needs. The recipes in this book can be used as-is, but are far more effective when customized to a specific skin type or hair type. No two people are exactly the same, which can make customizing recipes a challenge. When it comes to establishing your own routine, you are the best possible person for the job.

Find a balance that works for you. When it comes to natural beauty it's not all or nothing. Some people like to keep their hair care all-natural, but aren't ready to give up their favorite facial cream or commercial deodorant. That's okay! The two worlds don't have to be mutually exclusive. Any changes you choose to make will be worthwhile. While there are certain recipes that need to be used together (and I'll point those out as they come along), usually you can pick and choose which portions of your routine to keep all-natural. For example, you might choose to cleanse and condition your hair naturally, but continue to style your hair with commercial gel.

Be consistent. The recipes in this book are meant to help you create a whole new way of caring for your skin and hair. Repeatedly switching back and forth between handmade and commercial products is likely to wreak havoc—especially for those methods that involve a long adjustment period. Do yourself a favor, and do your best not to "cheat" on your natural routine.

ask a **NATURAL BEAUTY EXPERT**

Q: What inspired you to start making handmade and natural skin care products?

A: The more I learned about the power of foods to heal the body, the more I wanted to use some foods directly on my skin. I can see and feel the difference right away, so that kept the inspiration flowing.

Blythe Metz, BlytheNaturalLiving.com

ORGANIC VS. NATURAL

We hear the words *natural* and *organic* a lot—both in the grocery store and at the beauty counter. While both words have a similar definition in the dictionary, they have very different meanings when found on a label.

Organic is a term that the FDA uses to certify ingredients produced without chemicals or synthetic materials. Beauty products can be completely organic or they can be made with a combination of organic and conventional ingredients. Take a look at the ingredient listing to see how much of the product is actually organic.

The word *natural*, on the other hand, is not regulated by the FDA and is mostly used as a marketing term. It's generally accepted that a product marked as natural should contain only ingredients found in nature, but exactly how close to nature those ingredients are is open to interpretation. For example, a label might use the word natural to describe cocamide diethanolamine—a derivative of coconut which is just about as close to a coconut as a Jolly Rancher is to a watermelon.

When it comes to shopping for commercial beauty products, it's good to take the word natural with a grain of salt. In this book, *natural* indicates ingredients that are derived from natural sources, like plants.

BASIC TECHNIQUES

Most of the recipes in this book are as simple as mixing ingredients in a bowl or shaking them together in a bottle. There are two kinds of recipes that might be a little trickier to pull off. Emulsions (lotions and creams), and bar soap involve some extra steps and sometimes take practice to master. If these kinds of advanced recipes don't appeal to you, it's totally ok to cheat by purchasing a ready-made version of any of these basic natural products.

How to Make Lotions and Creams

Oils and waters don't usually mix, so it takes a little extra effort to create a mixture that uses both oil and water in one product. Lotions and creams are made using a technique called *emulsion*, which disperses water-based ingredients like water, hydrosol, or aloe gel into oils and fats. Emulsion might sound a bit intimidating, but it's actually a pretty simple process—one that's also used in the kitchen for salad dressings and sauces.

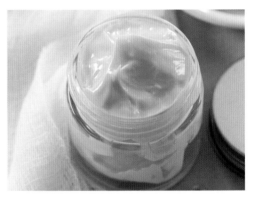

The trick to achieving a stable emulsion, one that won't separate as soon as it cools down, is to combine the water and oil phases at similar temperatures and then mix them really, really well. Emulsions need to be whisked continuously as they cool. If you try to skip those last few minutes of whisking, the emulsion may fail and leave you with a goopy mess instead of a smooth, creamy lotion.

TOXIC BEAUTY INGREDIENTS

Mineral Oil

Mineral oil is a byproduct of petroleum. While it is technically a natural ingredient made from natural minerals, it doesn't offer the same kind of moisturizing benefits found in high quality plant-based carrier oils. Whether or not mineral oil is actually toxic is uncertain, but there is limited data that links it to cancer and allergy and immune system disruption. Aside from possible risks, mineral oil offers very few benefits beyond being cheap and shelf stable—two qualities that cosmetic companies often value above all else.

How to Make Lotions and Creams (continued)

1 During the oil phase, combine the wax, butter and/or carrier oil in a double boiler, and heat until everything is fully melted together.

2 During the water phase warm the water-based ingredients in a small pan.

3 Do your best to make sure that the oil phase and water phase come to the same temperature.

4 Remove the oil phase from the heat and begin to whisk it. Pour the water phase into the oil phase in a slow, steady stream, whisking continuously as you do. An electric hand mixer comes in handy for larger batches.

5 Whisk the mixture for at least five minutes or for as long as it take to cool to room temperature. The mixture will thicken as it cools.

6 Stir in any essential oils that you may be using, then transfer the mixture to clean jars or bottles.

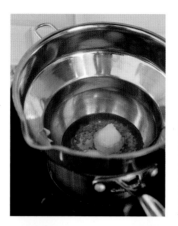
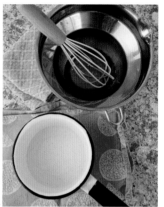
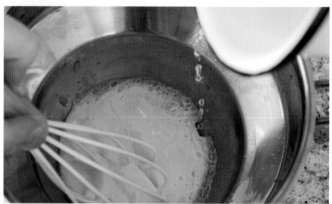
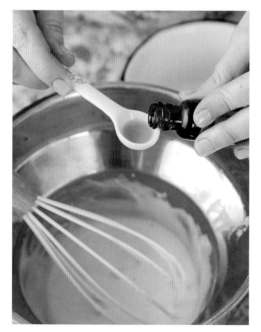
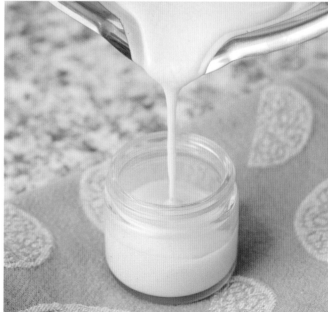

How to Make Hand-Milled Soap

Hand-milling is a great way for beginners to make their own customized, all-natural soaps. The process melts down pre-made soap with ingredients like oils, herbs, and clays, creating new bars that are totally customized—not to mention creamy, bubbly, and a pleasure to use.

In soap making circles, hand-milling is also called *rebatching* or *rebatch soap*. The process starts off by grating natural soap bars into shavings, then melting them down with liquids. Additives like carrier oils, herbs, and essential oils can be added to the melted soap in order to create custom recipes. Because the hand-milling process uses a relatively low heat it doesn't damage fragile ingredients the way that from-scratch soap making can. This makes hand-milling a great choice for specialty recipes like shampoo bars.

Start off with a high quality bar soap made with pure oils and butters. Castile soap is ideal because it is made from 100% olive oil. Some soap making suppliers even offer a rebatch base, a pre-shredded soap base made specifically for hand-milling. Avoid using commercial bar soap and melt-and-pour soap bases as these are made with totally different ingredients, making them unsuitable for the hand-milling process. It's also important to look for bar soap that doesn't contain salt. Salt is often added to natural soaps to harden the bars, but this makes them a real pain to melt down. Castile Bars from Vermont Soap, Austin Natural Soap, or castile rebatch base from Bramble Berry all work really well. (For contact information see the Resources section on page 122.)

You'll need a double boiler or a crockpot to make hand-milled soap. Direct heat will burn the soap, and it won't melt (or set back up) properly once it's been scorched. The soaps should be poured into molds made of wood or heat-proof silicone. Other kinds of molds may be too flimsy to handle hand-milled soap and could melt right along with the soap!

TOXIC BEAUTY INGREDIENTS

Fragrances

Did you know that there can be over one thousand components contained in a single ingredient marked as *fragrance*? Manufacturers aren't obligated to share their ingredients because their fragrance recipes are considered proprietary. This might not seem like a big deal until you learn more about the kinds of chemicals that can be found in fragrance. Studies have found some pretty nasty stuff—like neurotoxins, allergens, and sensitizers. Specific substances, like phthalates, get called out every now and then but for every ingredient that gets banned or drops out of use there could be many more right behind it. This explains why so many people find themselves sensitive to fragrances in body products, air fresheners, and laundry detergents.

How to Make Hand-Milled Soap (continued)

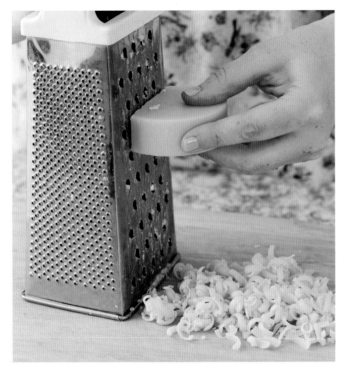

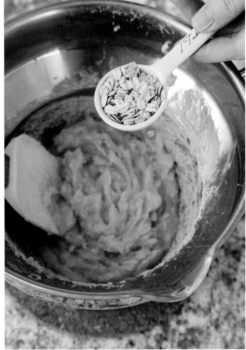

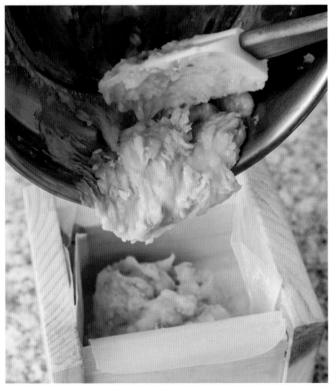

1 Grate the soap into shavings, then combine them in a double boiler or crock pot with liquid (water, beer, etc.).

2 Heat the soap and liquid until the ingredients are fully melted together. Be sure to stir the ingredients often.

3 Remove the ingredients from the heat. Stir in any additives while the mixture is still nice and hot.

4 Pour the melted soap into a silicone or wooden mold lined with wax paper. Allow the soap to cool until it is hard enough to handle. This can take anywhere from 1 to 3 days.

5 Once the soap has hardened, carefully remove it from the mold. If you used a large mold, now is the time to slice it into bars. Set the individual soaps on a drying rack and allow them to cure until fully dried and hardened. This can take anywhere from 1 to 3 weeks.

How to Apply a Facial Masque

While it's absolutely fine to slap homemade treatments on with reckless abandon, you might be surprised to learn that there is a proper way to apply a facial masque. Whether it's meant to cleanse, soothe, plump, or pamper, these simple application steps can help make the most of your facial.

1 Start off with bare skin that is free of any makeups or lotions.

2 Moisten a washcloth with hot water. It should be hot enough to generate steam, but not so hot that it will scald your face. Be careful not to burn your skin.

3 Drape the washcloth over your face. This will help open your pores, prepping your skin for your homemade treatment. Leave your skin damp or pat it dry according to the directions in your treatment.

4 Scoop the masque into the palm of one hand using a clean spoon or spatula. Using two fingers, gently spread the mixture onto your face in a slow, circular motion. Avoid your eyes, lips, and nostrils. You can also try applying on your masque with a clean paintbrush or makeup brush. Follow the recipe directions on how long to leave the masque on and how to remove it.

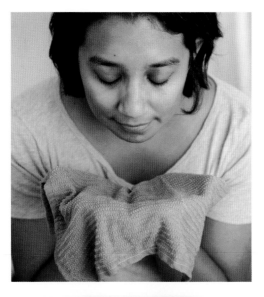

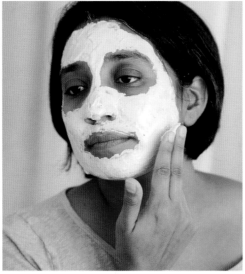

Masque Tips

Most masques can be left on for fifteen to thirty minutes. If your masque contains any drying or acidic ingredients like clay or lemon juice, be careful not to leave it on any longer than fifteen minutes.

If you find a homemade masque to be too slippery or wet, try adding a dry ingredient like oatmeal, oat flour, rice bran powder or adzuki bean powder.

Gentle masques can be used everyday, but any recipes that include drying or acidic ingredients like clay or lemon juice should be limited. Strong clays, like French green, green Illite, rhassoul, and multanni mitti (also known as fuller's earth) should be used once a week at most.

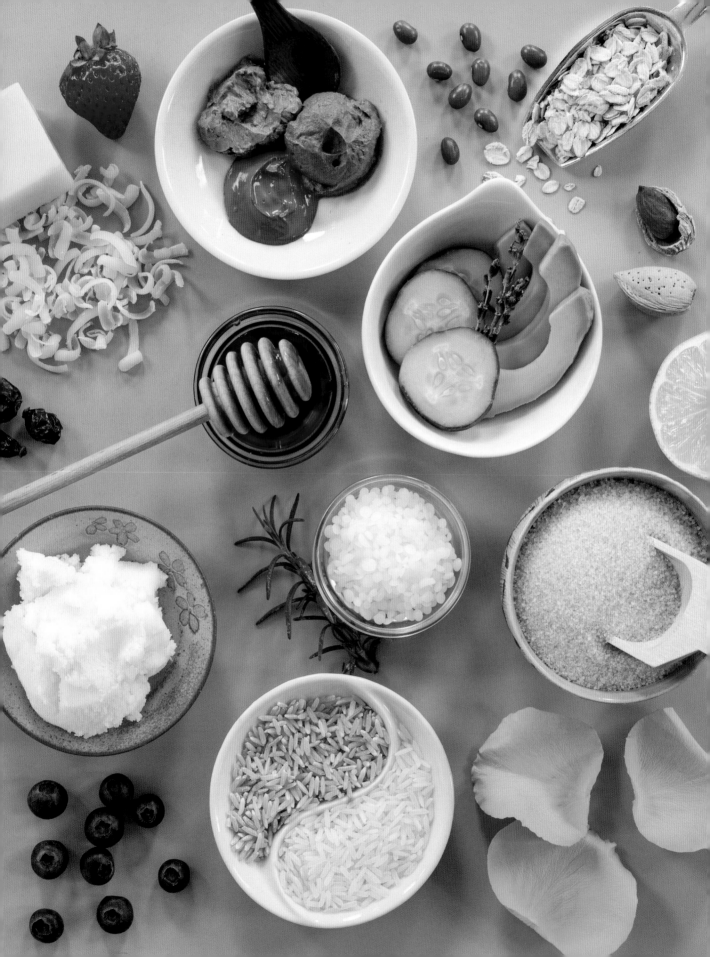

2

BUILDING YOUR PANTRY

It's easy to get carried away when it comes to building up an ingredient collection. With so many exotic oils and magical sounding herbs, you can easily find yourself amassing a horde of butters, serums, and elixirs. If you aren't careful, you may find yourself resembling a medieval apothecary rather than a green living guru. While it can be tempting to procure each and every exciting product that comes along, I recommend keeping your pantry simple, and customized to your own personal needs. Sure, you *could* end up needing that bottle of Amazonian sacha inchi oil one day, but you probably could have made do with something twice as common and half as expensive such as rose hip seed oil. The following chapter will highlight the most practical and commonly used ingredients for a natural beauty routine. »

STOCKING UP

THE IMPORTANCE OF QUALITY

It's important to remember that not all natural ingredients are created equally. Just because something is natural, doesn't mean that it was produced with cosmetic use in mind. Natural minerals are a great example of the importance of sourcing only cosmetic or food-grade ingredients (rather than industrial-grade) for your natural beauty routine.

While it is possible to harvest natural oxides from the earth, these raw minerals often contain heavy metals, such as lead and arsenic. While lead and arsenic are totally natural, you don't want them in your cosmetics. Raw minerals are often used for industrial purposes, while safer minerals are synthesized or purified in labs for cosmetic use.

Beeswax is another great example. Industrial beeswax is produced using much lower standards than cosmetic or food grade wax. It can include nasty pesticides and toxins, definitely not the kind of thing you would want to put in your lip balm.

SHOPPING SMART

With natural products growing in popularity, the market has become saturated with brick-and-mortar and online retailers offering ingredients for food and cosmetic use. These ingredients are imported from all corners of the world, sometimes with strict quality control standards, and sometimes not. Choose your suppliers wisely. Look for companies with well-established business histories and solid reputations for quality and customer service. Check out the list of recommended suppliers in the back of this book to get started.

It's important that the ingredients you are working with are pure, natural, and safe. Whenever possible, choosing *certified* organic ingredients is best, as the FDA imposes extra regulations and quality standards on certified organic ingredients. Never buy an ingredient that you aren't sure is either cosmetic or food grade, and always purchase directly from trusted suppliers or local artisans. If you're unsure about the quality or nature of an ingredient, ask questions. Your supplier should always be able to provide you with the INCI (international nomenclature of cosmetic ingredients) or the scientific name and ingredient listing for any products they sell. You can also request documentation, such as certificates of analysis, from most trustworthy suppliers.

INGREDIENT STORAGE AND SHELF LIFE

Natural cosmetic ingredients should be treated with the same care as the food in your kitchen. Like food, ingredients like vegetable butter, grain powders, and carrier oils will eventually expire. Rancidity or oxidation can occur quickly when ingredients are exposed to air, light, moisture, or extreme temperatures.

As a rule, dry powders should be stored in airtight containers in a cool, dry place. Fats, like carrier oils and vegetable butters can be stored in sealed containers at room temperature for several months or in the refrigerator for long-term storage. Fragile ingredients with shelf lives of six months or less should always be refrigerated.

Keep a close eye on your ingredients for signs of spoilage. If the ingredients change in color, texture, or aroma, it may be a sign that they've gone rancid. Rancid ingredients can change pH level, becoming more acidic over time, and thus damaging to your skin. The nutrients and benefits of natural ingredients can also diminish over time, which is why, like food, natural cosmetics are best made in small batches with fresh ingredients. Purchasing ingredients in small quantities will help keep your stock fresh and potent.

FAQ

What are the Differences Between Ingredient Classifications?

Organic Ingredients

- Sourced from growers and manufacturers certified by the USDA National Organic Program
- Produced without the use of prohibited substances such as chemical pesticides and fertilizers
- Both food-grade and cosmetic-grade ingredients may also be certified as Organic

Food Grade Ingredients

- Edible ingredients, both fresh and packaged
- Produced and packaged using food-grade standard set by the FDA
- Can be eaten or used in skin care and hair care products

Cosmetic Grade Ingredients

- Cosmetics and soap making supplies such as clays, grains, essential oils, vegetable butters, etc.
- Produced and packaged using cosmetic-grade standards set by the FDA
- Can be used in skin care and hair care products but should not be eaten

Industrial Grade Ingredients

- Produced for use in industrial products such as paint, building, and machinery.
- Should never be used in food, skin care, or hair care products.

THE ESSENTIAL INGREDIENTS

ADZUKI BEAN POWDER

A traditional Japanese beauty ingredient, this finely milled bean powder gently exfoliates the skin without drying it out. Adzuki bean powder can be used on its own with plain water to create a simple and effective daily cleanser. It can also be blended with cosmetic clays, almond flour, yogurt, carrier oils, and other natural ingredients to create specialty masques and treatments.

ALMONDS

Finely milled almond flour makes a great exfoliant. It's gentle enough for facial cleansers, but sturdy enough for body scrubs and masques too. Almonds are also rich in calcium and magnesium, both minerals that can help skin appear brighter and more healthy.

ALOE VERA GEL

Aloe vera is famous for its soothing, anti-inflammatory properties. It can be used as-is to soothe bug bites, sunburn, or mild skin irritations. Aloe vera gel makes a great substitute for water in toners, lotions, creams, and masques. It can even be used in hair sprays and body spritzes. Also known as aloe vera juice, pure aloe vera gel has a thin, water-like consistency. Steer clear of aloe vera products with jelly-like textures, as these probably contain undesirable additives. When in doubt, check the label on the packaging. Aloe vera should be the only ingredient listed.

APPLE CIDER VINEGAR

In addition to being an excellent ingredient in salad dressings, apple cider vinegar is a natural beauty VIP. Buy raw, organic, and unfiltered apple cider vinegar when you can, as this will be by far the most potent type available. When properly diluted, apple cider vinegar helps to balance skin's pH, disinfect and tame troublesome bacteria, and soothe itchy, irritated skin. It is an essential part of any natural hair care routine, and acts as both a conditioner and detangler. In skin care, diluted apple cider vinegar makes an excellent toner.

BAKING SODA

Sodium bicarbonate, better known as baking soda, is a household staple that doubles as an indispensable ingredient for any natural beauty routine. Baking soda is naturally alkaline, while the mixture of sweat and sebum that collects on your skin and hair is acidic. The reaction between these two substances allows baking soda to gently cleanse and exfoliate without stripping your skin and hair.

[A] lavender buds

[B] turbinado sugar

[C] sea clay

[D] rose clay

[E] almond flour

[F] sea salt

[G] oatmeal

[H] brown rice

[I] white rice

[J] rice bran flour

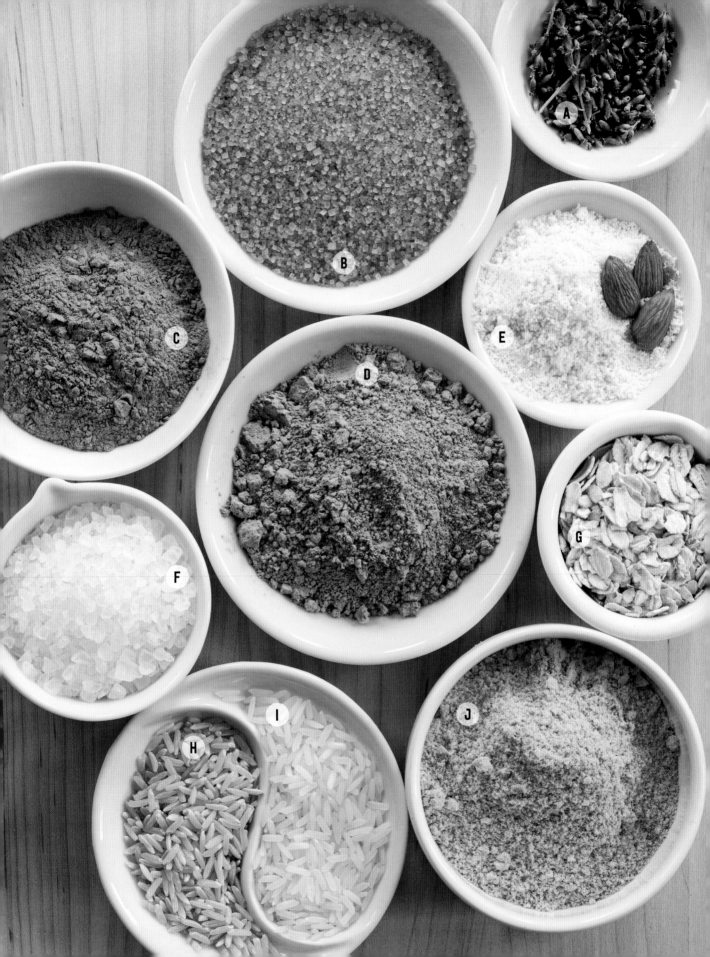

BEESWAX AND CANDELILLA WAX

Wax is used to harden balms and salves. It is also use as a main ingredient in emulsions, such as lotions and creams. The two most commonly used waxes for natural skin care are beeswax and candelilla wax. Beeswax is the most common and easiest to use, having a relatively soft and pliable texture. Candelilla is a better choice for vegans, or those who prefer not to use animal-based ingredients. It has a much harder texture, so recipes often need to be adjusted to compensate for that. To make vegan creams and lotions, you can use either candelilla wax or emulsifying wax instead of beeswax.

CARRIER OILS

There are about as many carrier oils for natural skin care and hair care as there are stars in the sky. Before you get too overwhelmed by the possibilities, keep in mind that you only need a few favorites to accompany a simple beauty routine.

Organic Virgin Coconut Oil:
The rich, decadent aroma of this oil will make it very hard to resist. While I am often tempted to slather myself in this oil from head to toe, I use just a few dabs as an extra conditioner whenever I wash my hair. Organic virgin coconut oil is moisturizing, but also astringent. Its light texture is great for everyday hair care and skin care.

Clockwise from top: rose hip seed oil, watermelon seed oil, tamanu oil.

Rose Hip Seed Oil: This highly moisturizing oil is as light as a feather and packed with antioxidants, making it an excellent base for a facial serums and creams. Rose hip seed oil can also be used as an additive in facial masques, body oils, and oil-cleansers.

Castor Oil: Castor oil is very thick and greasy. It may not seem like the kind of thing that you would want to put on your face, but it is a key ingredient for the oil cleansing method. It's also a good choice for foot care. Castor oil is too greasy for use as a moisturizing ingredient on the rest of your body.

Watermelon Seed Oil: This miracle oil has a very pleasant texture that is non-greasy, and easily absorbed into the skin. Watermelon seed oil is an excellent ingredient to have on hand for almost any recipe, including scrubs, lotions, balms, body butters, and hair conditioners. Watermelon seed oil is relatively inexpensive compared to other specialty oils with similar properties, so I recommend keeping a good amount handy for general use.

Apricot Kernel Oil: Another excellent oil for daily use, apricot kernel oil is sometimes easier to find than watermelon seed oil. It makes a great base for almost any recipe, and can be used in both skin and hair care products.

Avocado Oil: This carrier oil is thicker and heavier than watermelon seed oil, but not nearly as greasy as castor oil, making it the perfect choice for adding extra conditioning power to recipes meant for dry skin or dry hair.

Jojoba: Scientifically speaking, jojoba is actually not an oil but a liquid wax. This unique ingredient mimics your skin's natural sebum almost exactly. Sebum is the natural lubricant and protectant your body produces for the hair and skin. For this reason, Jojoba makes a great moisturizer, but just like sebum, jojoba oil can clog your skin if used too heavily.

Clockwise from top left: pink kaolin clay, dry; pink kaolin clay, wet, sea clay, wet; sea clay, dry.

COSMETIC GRADE CLAY

Clay has the amazing ability to draw out dirt, toxins, and oils from your skin. This makes it an excellent ingredient for cleansers, masques, and even detoxifying baths. Because these ingredients are mineral-based, it is very important to make sure that you only purchase cosmetic grade clay. Industrial clays can contain dangerous heavy metals, such as lead and arsenic.

Different varieties of clay possess varying strengths, some drawing out much more moisture than others. Keep your skin type in mind when choosing the right clays for your pantry. Following, you will find explanations of the different types of clay used in beauty products.

- Kaolin is the most gentle family of clays, white kaolin, being the mildest of all. Kaolin can be used on all skin types. Even children and those with sensitive skin can use kaolin clay.

- Sea clay and Dead Sea clay are a bit stronger, and should be used with more caution. Those with oily skin can use these daily, but others should limit the application of sea clay to weekly masques or occasional treatments.

- The strongest clays are French green, green Illite, rhassoul, and multanni mitti (also known as fuller's earth). These clays should be limited to one application per week, and should only be used by those with oily skin.

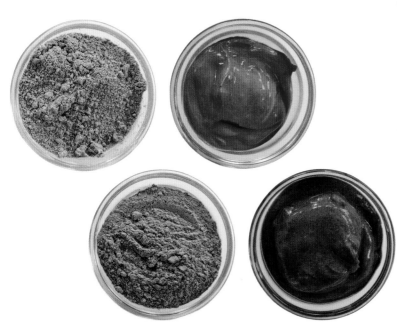

ESSENTIAL OILS

Essential oils are highly potent, steam-distilled plant extracts. Though completely natural, they must be handled and used with care. Essential oils are used medicinally by aromatherapists. Like any medicine, these natural chemicals can be harmful if used improperly. It's important to research any essential oil before using it in your routine. You'll need to determine its recommended dilution, and check to see if the oil has any restrictions for use. Certain essential oils can be disruptive to medical conditions like pregnancy, high blood pressure, or epilepsy.

As a rule, any essential oil you are working with should be diluted to around 1–3% for use in skin care. That means that the oil needs to be blended with a carrier oil to be used directly, or used in very small proportions in recipes and formulations.

It's important to note that essential oils should be used with extreme care on children and babies. Kids and babies can't process the chemicals in essential oils as easily as adults. If you are pregnant, I recommend consulting a doctor or aromatherapist before using or handling any essential oils. Check out the Resources page to find websites that offer more information on essential oil safety. While there are thousands of essential oils available, I tend to lean on a handful of favorites. Choose one or two that suit your skin type, and invest in small bottles of high quality oil.

Rose Essential Oil: The ultimate oil for mature skin care, rose essential oil is treasured for its ability to help soothe and soften. Rose essential oil is soothing to all skin types, and is an excellent addition to any of your most precious facial recipes.

Geranium Essential Oil: Geranium essential oil makes a great alternative to rose essential oil and is far less expensive. It can still help balance skin pH, fight fine lines and wrinkles, and benefit facial recipes. Though any variety of geranium essential oil will do, my personal favorites are rose geranium and geranium bourbon.

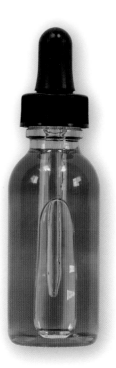

Essential oils should always be stored in glass or stainless steel containers. These potent ingredients can dissolve plastic and eat through rubber.

FAQ

Should My Ingredients Be Organic?

Purchasing organic ingredients for skin care whenever possible is ideal if you can manage it. If not, keep in mind that some ingredients carry a heavier load of pesticides, antibiotics, and other nasty bits than others. If you pick and choose which items to buy organic, go with fresh dairy, berries, and soft fruits. Carrier oils, butters, and other ingredients come in organic varieties, but choosing organic with these ingredients may not be as crucial. If prices are comparable, go for it. But if choosing organic pushes natural beauty beyond your budget, stick with conventional ingredients. Like shopping for groceries, the decision between buying organic and conventional ingredients comes down to personal preference.

FAQ

Will I Save Money Using a Natural Routine?

That really depends on how much you are already spending on store-bought products. Considering that a bottle of shampoo can cost anywhere from one dollar to over twenty dollars, it's safe to say that the cost comparison will vary from person to person. That being said, most of the ingredients in these recipes are relatively affordable, with the exception of certain essential oils or carrier oils that come a bit more dear. Replacing your products one at a time is a good way to keep the cost of switching to a natural routine easier to manage. If you were to buy all the ingredients listed in this book at once, you'd be looking at a pretty hefty price tag.

Neroli Essential Oil: Neroli essential oil is another great choice for facial care. Like rose essential oil and geranium essential oil, it helps to balance skin's moisture. Which of the three you choose mostly depends on budget and personal preference. Personally, I adore the smell of neroli essential oil. It is made from orange blossoms, giving it a delightfully sweet and floral scent.

Roman Chamomile Essential Oil: Roman chamomile essential oil is very effective at soothing itchy, red skin. It also has a calming effect emotionally, which as far as side effects go, is not too shabby.

Yarrow Essential Oil: Another great essential oil for soothing inflamed skin, yarrow is also slightly astringent, making it a good choice for oily or combination skin.

Helichrysum Essential Oil: Helichrysum essential oil is expensive, but a worthwhile investment for those fighting acne. It not only possesses potent antibacterial and antifungal properties, it can help reduce scarring. Helichrysum essential oil's restorative properties also make it a good choice for mature skin.

Niaouli Essential Oil: Niaouli essential oil is a close relative to tea tree essential oil, an ingredient commonly used to combat acne. While both boast potent antibacterial properties and are excellent for acne-prone and combination skin, niaouli essential oil is more gentle on the nervous system and overall health. I recommend using niaouli essential oil in place of tea tree essential oil in recipes.

Peppermint Essential Oil: I use peppermint essential oil in almost all of my lip balm recipes. The hint of cooling mint will make your lips tingle. That stimulating feeling can also benefit tired muscles in your feet, legs, and hands. A word to the wise though: a little peppermint essential oil goes a long way, so go easy with this particular essential oil. By the way, do not use peppermint essential oil with babies or toddlers.

Rosemary Essential Oil: Rosemary is a popular essential oil in haircare recipes because it encourages a healthy balance of oils in the scalp. It is believed to discourage dandruff, soothe inflammation, and may even stimulate hair growth.

EGGS

As far as old wives' tales go, slathering one's head in mayonnaise to get gorgeous, shining locks, is actually not a bad idea. The cholesterol contained in eggs can help reinforce damaged hair, and its natural lecithin provides shine and luster. While the mayonnaise in your refrigerator does contain some of these benefits, a fresh-made emulsion of organic eggs, nutritive carrier oil, and apple cider vinegar is so much better. You can even dress up this homemade hair mayo with a beneficial essential oil.

FRUITS AND VEGETABLES

I love using fresh produce in homemade skin care treatments. Keep in mind that whenever you incorporate fresh ingredients, like fruits, veggies, herbs, and dairy products, your recipes should be used up right away. Sometimes you can get away with storing leftovers in the fridge for a few days. Generally, these kinds of recipes are best when fresh.

Berries: Strawberries, raspberries, and blackberries are packed with alpha-hydroxy acids. These gentle acids help dissolve sebum, and slough off dead skin cells, making skin look glowing and bright.

Banana: Mashed banana contains a lot of vitamin B, which can help reduce redness and inflammation. Use bananas in soothing and moisturizing masques. Banana"s high potassium levels can also help balance your skin's pH level.

FAQ

Are the Recipes in this Book Edible?

While most of the ingredients used in this book are technically edible, you probably wouldn't want to eat them. For one thing, cosmetic ingredient suppliers are seldom set up to repackage their products as food grade. While the practices used to handle cosmetics are perfectly safe, they aren't held to the same standards as facilities licensed to handle food. Certain ingredients, like essential oils, clay, and castile soap—really shouldn't be eaten, anyway. If you find yourself getting hungry while reading this book, head for the kitchen—not your skin care stash.

Cucumber: We've all seen ladies in spa commercials relaxing with cucumber slices over their eyes. Cucumbers are great for soothing skin because they are naturally cooling and anti-inflammatory. Cucumber contains a bounty of antioxidant and is mildly astringent, meaning it can help to balance skin's moisture levels. Cucumbers are a classic ingredient for masques, but they can also be used to reduce puffiness and increase circulation anywhere on your body.

Fresh Herbs: You can kick up your masques and scrubs by including pureed herbs. Spearmint, chamomile, and marigold can be added to soothing recipes for their cooling and anti-inflammatory benefits. Herbs like basil, lavender, and lemon balm can be used to help fight acne.

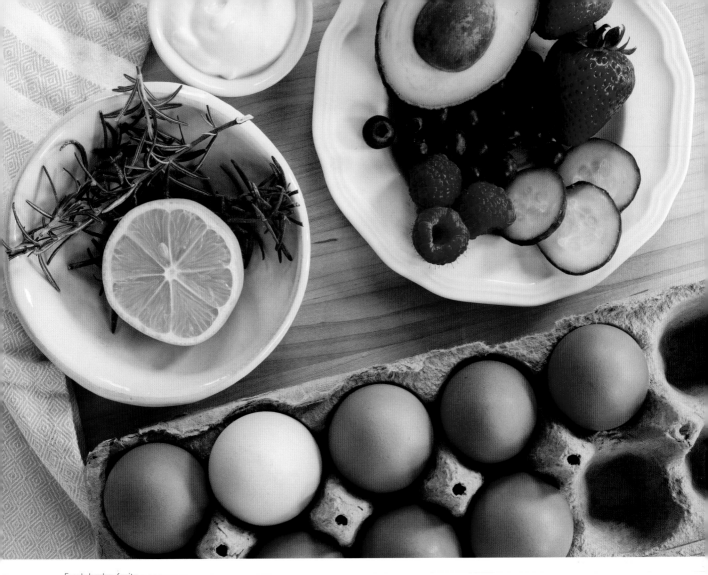

Fresh herbs, fruits, vegetables, and dairy products contain active ingredients that can be highly beneficial in homemade beauty products.

HONEY

One of nature's most amazing wonder-foods, honey contains natural antibacterial, anti-inflammatory, and antifungal properties. This makes it an excellent tool for skin care. Honey can be used to cleanse, soothe, and heal troubled skin. It's unique combination of soothing and healing properties makes it especially beneficial to combination skin types. Those with normal, sensitive, or acne-prone skin can also benefit from the inclusion of honey in soaps, cleansers, and masques.

HYDROSOLS

Hydrosols are a byproduct that is created when essential oils are made. Essential oils are steam distilled. When a batch is completed, the leftover steam is collected and bottled as hydrosol. Like essential oils, hydrosols contain natural chemicals that can be used to benefit beauty and aromatherapy treatments. However, hydrosols are much milder than essential oils, and can be used more liberally than their potent counterparts.

Don't be surprised if the hydrosols you use don't smell exactly how you might

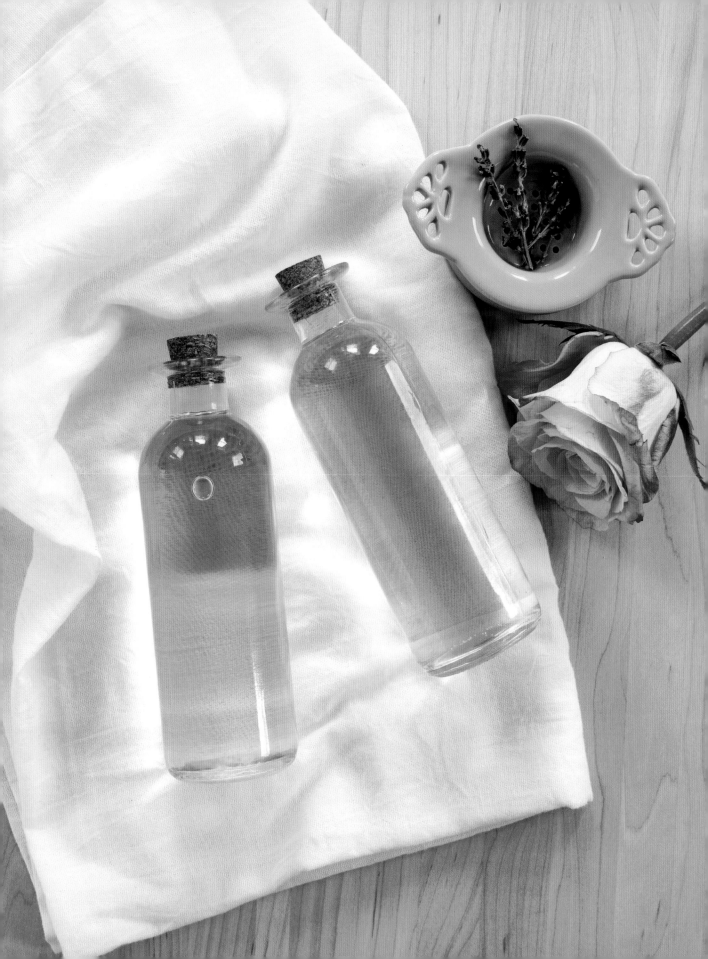

expect. These water-based distillations are very diluted, and the most recognizable scents from the plants used to make them often end up in their twin essential oils instead. Hydrosols make excellent toners and are fabulous in masques, cleansers, and rinses. Try to keep one or two types that that correspond to your skin and beauty routine.

Rose or Rose Geranium Hydrosol: If you invest in only one hydrosol, make it rose. Rose water is a classic beauty ingredient for good reason. It can be used from head to toe and is especially beneficial to mature skin. If rose hydrosol is too pricey, look for rose geranium hydrosol instead. It tends to be less expensive and can replace rose.

Chamomile or Yarrow Hydrosol: Both of these hydrosols are perfect for soothing itchy, irritated, or inflamed skin. They work well for dry skin, combination skin, or conditions like eczema or psoriasis.

Neroli Hydrosol: This particular hydrosol is a luxury, pure and simple. It has a beautiful aroma, and like rose hydrosol, can help to balance skin and lift spirits.

Witch Hazel or Lavender Hydrosol: If you have acne prone skin or combination skin, keeping a hydrosol on hand with disinfecting properties is a good idea. Both lavender and witch hazel hydrosols contain both antibacterial and anti-inflammatory properties, making them not only healing, but also soothing.

Most carrier oils can be used directly on the skin and hair to provide instant moisture. Hydrosols make excellent toners, body sprays, and hair spritzes.

RICE BRAN POWDER OR RICE FLOUR

Rice bran powder and rice flour are gentle, non-drying exfoliants and are often easier to find than adzuki bean powder. They can be mixed with water or hydrosol for use as a cleanser or added to masques, scrubs, and other recipes for cleansing or exfoliating your skin.

SEA SALT AND RAW SUGAR

With salt and sugar, nature has provided two of the most perfect body exfoliants. Look for a fine to medium grain size for scrubs, body polishes, and most any other skincare recipe. In addition to being an excellent exfoliant, sea salt contains a bounty of healthy minerals that can help improve skin's circulation and soothe skin conditions like eczema and psoriasis. Raw sugar also contains healthy mineral content and provides gentle exfoliation for sensitive or irritated skin. Raw sugar can also be used to create DIY hair removal treatments.

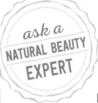

ask a NATURAL BEAUTY EXPERT

Q: Which ingredients do you use most in your DIY routine? Do you have a favorite?

A: I cannot live without honey, lemon, and sea salt. They are three of my favorite things. I always like to add these ingredients whenever I can. Not only are these ingredients great, but most people already have them in their home. They just fix everything!

Narae Kim, Artifactgirl.com

SOY LECITHIN

Lecithin is a thick, gooey substance that is often used as an additive in not only skin care ingredients, but also junk food. You may recognize the scent of lecithin from the suspiciously soft and pliable caramel in candy bars. While lecithin is great for assisting natural emulsions and improving the texture and adhesion in lip balms, you won't catch me taking a bite. Lecithin is used in very small quantities in skin care recipes.

UNSCENTED, DYE-FREE COLD PROCESS SOAP

Soap can be a champion in recipes because it can grab on to water and oil at the same time. Soap encapsulates dirt, bacteria, and oil, and then rinses it away. It's the best way to remove dangerous bacteria from skin without harming the helpful microorganisms. Soap is a useful ingredient in a number of basic skin care and hair care recipes, so I always keep a bit of natural, unscented, cold process soap on hand.

Cold process soap is made by saponifying raw oils and fats with lye and water. Though lye is extremely caustic, it evaporates from the soap as it cures. Cold process soap can be made in an endless variety of recipes, and can include both natural and synthetic ingredients. For your pantry, look for an all-natural, unscented soap. Castile, a traditional olive-based soap, is ideal for building other recipes. It can be purchased or handmade in both bar and liquid form.

VEGETABLE BUTTERS

Vegetable butters are far thicker and heavier than carrier oils, and are used to provide intense moisture to body and skin care recipes. While most vegetable butters are too thick for facial use, they are excellent ingredients for lip care, foot care, dry hair types, and all-over body care. Like carrier oils, there are plenty to choose from, but a few favorites will suffice in building a well-stocked beauty pantry.

Shea Butter: This classic beauty ingredient comes in several varieties. Raw shea butter is touted as the most effective, but it has a very strong aroma that doesn't sit well with everyone. Refined shea butter is nearly odorless and colorless, and tends to be easier to work with than raw shea butter. If possible, try to get your hands on organic shea butter, or better yet, organic nilotica shea butter, a particularly rich and creamy variety that I adore.

Cocoa Butter: Pure cocoa butter has a very characteristic aroma that you will

[A] natural bar soap

[B] white beeswax

[C] yellow beeswax

[D] candelilla wax

[E] emulsifying wax

[F] cacao beans

[G] cocoa butter

[H] organic virgin coconut cream oil

[I] shea butter

[J] castile bar soap, whole and shredded

FAQ

Should I Be Concerned About Allergies?

Consider allergies before working with particular natural ingredients. If you have a nut allergy, for instance, you may have a reaction to sweet almond oil or even shea butter, which also comes from a nut. Those with latex allergies may be sensitive to shea or cocoa butter, which contain natural latex proteins. When in doubt, consult an allergist.

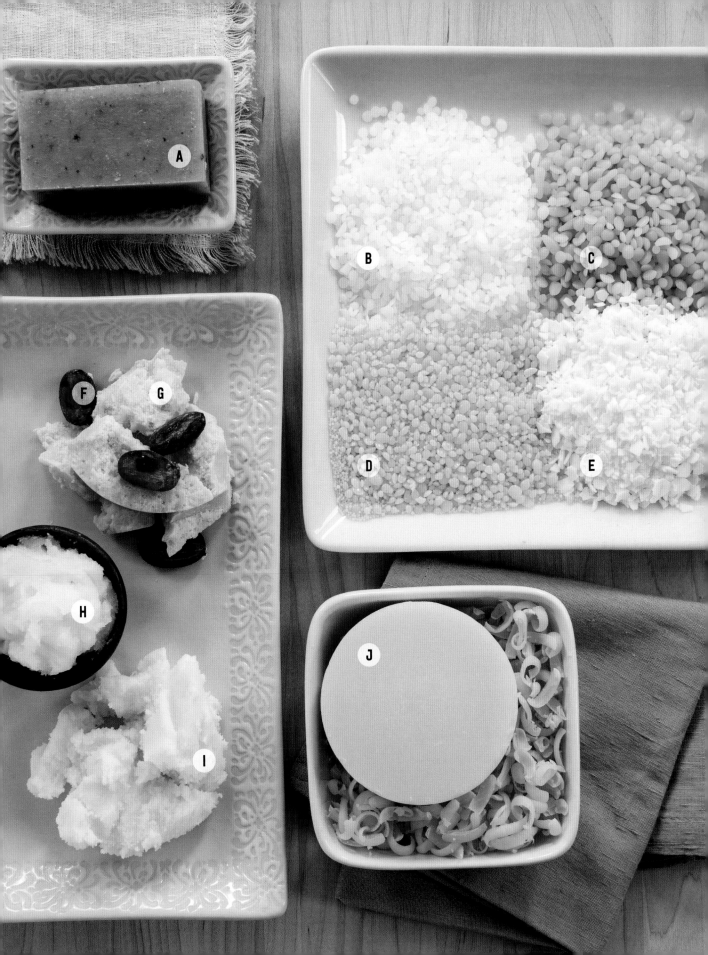

instantly recognize as the rich, creamy chocolate of your dreams. This super-hard butter is an intense conditioner, but a bit on the greasy side. While cocoa butter can certainly be enjoyed as-is, I usually like to blend it with something lighter, like watermelon seed oil or shea butter.

WITCH HAZEL

Witch hazel is a water soluble extract derived from a plant valued for its medicinal properties. It makes an excellent toner and wetting agent for masques and cleansers, having both soothing and astringent properties. Witch hazel can also help disinfect the skin, making it ideal for combination or acne-prone skin types. Witch hazel is most commonly available in an alcohol base. That variety works fine, but can be a bit drying. If you can find it. try using witch hazel hydrosol, which is usually alcohol-free.

YOGURT

You might remember the old stories of bathing beauty queens in buttermilk before a big pageant. Lactic acid, which is found in milk, yogurt, and other dairy products, can help to brighten dull skin by gently exfoliating dead cells from your skin's surface. Soaking in milk is actually an excellent way to smooth, soften, and polish your skin. There are few exfoliants as gentle or as soothing as dairy.

My top choice for homemade beauty recipes is plain, full-fat organic yogurt. The thick consistency and active cultures make it a wonderful masque as-is. It can also be mixed with mashed berries, cosmetic clays and herbs to create masques, body scrubs, and cleansers.

BORAX

Borax is a synthetic ingredient, but it's necessary for creating stable emulsions in natural lotion and cream recipes. It's a type of mineral salt technically named sodium borate, and it's used to soften the waters in lotion recipes in order to reduce surface tension and encourage emulsion. Basically, borax helps make sure that handmade creams and lotions don't separate after they cool. While you can sometimes get a handmade emulsion to work without borax, its absence makes the process much more fussy and unpredictable. If you are opposed to using borax, another alternative for easy emulsion is to replace the beeswax, lecithin, and borax in these recipes with emulsifying wax. Emulsifying wax is a plant-based wax that contains a special alcohol to aid in stabilizing lotion and creams recipes.

CHOOSING THE RIGHT INGREDIENTS FOR YOUR OWN ROUTINE

While this list might seem awfully long, keep in mind that you'll only need to invest in the ingredients that match your skin type and routine. Everyone's skin and hair is slightly different, which is why creating your own customized beauty routine can have such wonderful effects.

When you are getting ready to use the recipes in this book, refer back to this chapter to find the ingredients that will suit you best. If you aren't sure which to pick, I recommend choosing the ingredients best suited to sensitive or mature skin. Those ingredients tend to work well for everyone.

It can also help to purchase small quantities of ingredients when you first get started. Natural beauty can sometimes require experimentation. You may need to try a few different ingredients before discovering your favorite. Try to embrace this particular part of the challenge by allowing yourself to have fun and be creative.

FAQ

What kind of tools and equipment do I need to get started?

Most recipes in this book can be made with nothing more than a spoon and mixing bowl, but there are a few that require extra tools.

- A **double boiler** is a special kind of pot that allows ingredients to melt at a lower temperature than they would in a regular saucepan. Using one is the best way to melt butters, waxes, and solid oils as the lower heat won't damage the ingredients.
- Having a **blender** or a **food processor** handy helps make mixing up fresh masques as easy as making a smoothie.
- An **electric hand-mixer** takes the pain out of whipping up body butters, creams, and lotions that require extended whisking.
- If you get into soap making, you'll need a **sturdy metal grater** and a wooden or silicone **soap mold.**
- **Pipette droppers** are great for dispensing small amounts of essential oils into handmade recipes. Tiny droppers can be purchased online from most craft or soap making supply sites.
- Collecting **small bottles, jars,** and **canisters** to hold your handmade products can be as much fun as making them. Look for small containers in food or cosmetic grade plastic, glass, and stainless steel.

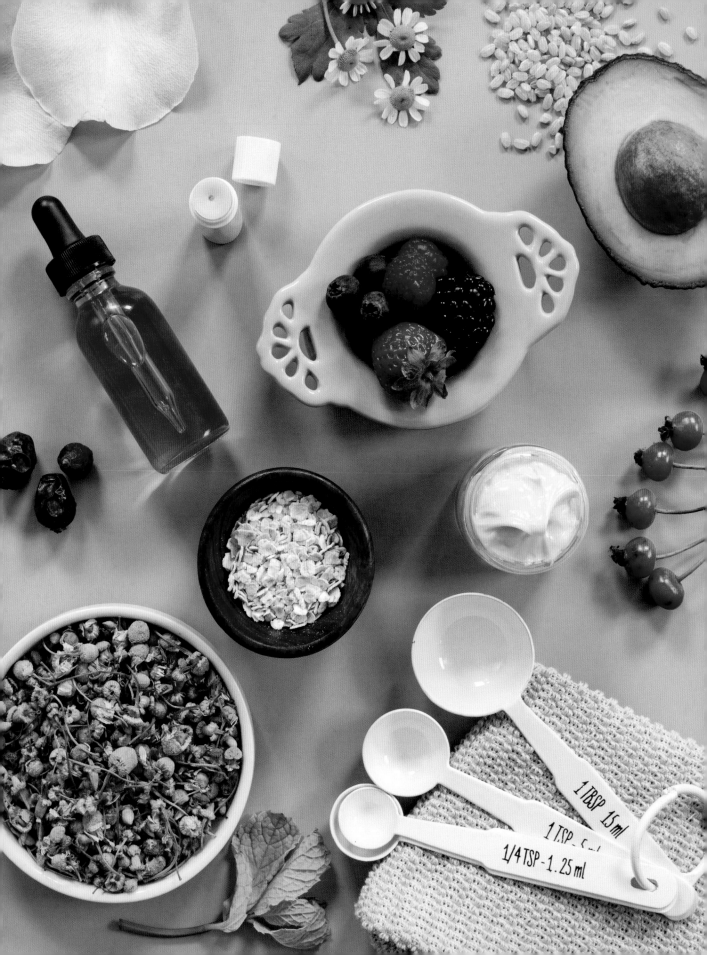

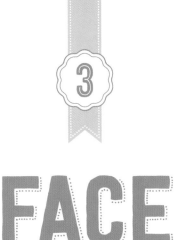

FACE

As far as beauty goes, facial care is pretty high on the priority list. Who hasn't wrestled with issues like acne, dryness, or irritation? While there are hundreds, if not thousands, of commercial products out there that promise relief from these common skin care challenges, the ingredients used in these products often do more to exacerbate the issues than help. Harsh detergents like sodium laurel sulfate and chemical-based additives, like silicone and parabens can leave skin irritated and with an unbalanced pH. Luckily, replacing your commercial facial care products can be surprisingly simple. In fact, facial care is usually the first area that I recommend for switching over to a totally natural and do-it-yourself routine. Simple cleansers and natural moisturizers made from whole ingredients can help your skin learn to balance itself naturally.

A basic natural beauty routine should consist of an everyday cleanser, a toner, and a moisturizer. These three products are all you really need to keep your skin looking great on a regular basis. Adding special recipes, like masques and facial » treatments is a great way to take your skin care regimen one step further. I'd recommend starting your transition to an all-natural routine by replacing your cleanser first, followed by your toner, then your moisturizer. Transitioning in steps will give your skin time to adjust while making the process less overwhelming for you as well.

GETTING STARTED

Determining the approach to natural skin care for your particular skin type will involve a little trial and error. It takes time and practice to identify the natural ingredients and perfect a technique that works best for your skin. It's important to keep in mind that different parts of your body may have different skin types. Someone could have a dry scalp, oily skin on their back, and combination skin on their face.

This chapter features two different methods for both cleansing and moisturizing the skin on your face. The first is an overview of the Oil Cleansing Method, which uses carrier oils to remove sebum from within the pores. The second offers exfoliation through use of a simple grain-based scrub. I recommend giving each method a try before settling on your favorite. And don't be afraid to experiment! If something isn't working for you, swap out an ingredient and try it again.

Once you settle into a natural routine that suits you well, your skin should respond by becoming clearer, less prone to redness, and better able to regulate its own moisture levels. You also will have the comfort of knowing that you are no longer exposing your body to toxic dyes, preservatives, and additives. Looking better and feeling better—what's not to love?

WHAT TO EXPECT

Even once you find the best recipe and method for your needs, you may go through an adjustment period while your skin gets used to the new routine. Part of what makes natural skin care great is that the gentle ingredients help your skin relearn how to keep itself well-conditioned. It can take time for your skin to learn exactly how much sebum to produce once it is no longer stripped by harsh detergents on a daily basis. At first you may experience an overproduction of oil or a period of dryness. For this reason, give a new skin care method two to three weeks before deciding whether or not it works for you.

PERSONAL STORIES

Is My Face Red?

I've battled redness and irritation since I was a teenager. Before I started my natural skincare routine I spent a small fortune on products marketed for sensitive skin. No matter what I tried, the redness never faded and I began to believe that I was destined to spend the rest of my life piling on makeup to try to hide my splotchy skin. It wasn't until I discovered adzuki bean powder that I saw a real improvement. By cutting out the harsh detergents in even the most benign commercial face washes I ended the cycle of over-drying and aggravating my sensitive skin. When I added a facial oil with anti-inflammatory and antibacterial ingredients, my skin began to clear up completely.

THE OIL CLEANSING METHOD

If washing your face with oil sounds crazy to you, don't worry—you are not alone. The commercial beauty industry has put a lot of effort into making oil sound like the enemy. Oil-free cleansers and moisturizers are extremely popular as a result.

Considering that soap-based cleansers are meant to remove oil from your skin, adding oil to get your face clean seems totally counterintuitive. Despite how wacky this concept may sound at first, the oil-cleansing method actually works really well for most people!

The method is founded on the concept that like removes like. Soap and detergents can scour the surface of your skin, removing every last drop of moisture (including the good stuff) but they have a hard time reaching beneath the surface, into your skin's pores, where excess sebum and bacteria can build up. Those clogged pores can result in acne, redness, uneven skin texture, or even infections. Oil, on the other hand, can dissolve the sebum in those backed up pores, keeping them healthy and clean.

Of course, you can't use just any oil with this method. Castor oil, a thick and gooey carrier oil, acts as the base for all oil-cleansing recipes. This super-greasy and sticky oil does a great job of grabbing on to excess dirt and oil—maybe too great of a job. Castor oil's intensity is mellowed out by being blended with light, moisturizing carrier oils, such as rosehip seed oil, watermelon oil, or avocado oil. You can customize your oil cleanser by choosing a carrier oil that suits your skin type, and by adjusting the ratio of castor oil in the blend.

It's important to note that though this cleanser is made entirely of oil, in some cases it can leave the skin feeling quite dry. Other users find that their skin remains perfectly moisturized after oil cleansing. I always recommend following any cleanser with a toner. Toners help balance the skin's pH and remove any leftover residue the cleanser may leave behind. Using a moisturizer is totally optional—especially with the oil cleansing method. You may also find that you don't need to use this cleanser on a daily basis. Unless you wear makeup, using the cleanser two or three times per week is often more than enough. On off days, simply rinse your face with warm water.

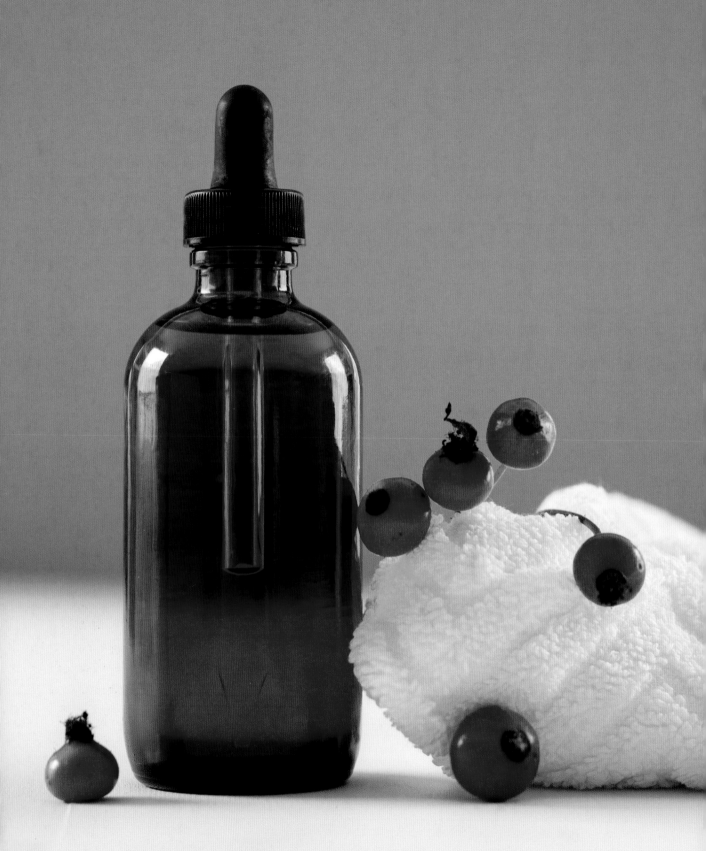

everyday recipe

OIL CLEANSERS

These basic oil cleanser recipes can be customized by adjusting the ratio of castor oil to other carrier oils. The more castor oil the recipe contains the more aggressive its cleansing power. For a less-drying blend, reduce the amount of castor oil. You can also swap out the other carrier oils with specialty ingredients that are well-suited to your skin type.

	MATURE SKIN	ACNE-PRONE SKIN	SENSITIVE SKIN
Optional Add-Ons	Argan Oil Evening Primrose Oil Pomegranate Seed Oil	Neem Oil Perilla Seed	Oat Oil Raspberry Seed Oil Tamanu Oil

INGREDIENTS

For normal skin:

- 2 tablespoons castor oil
- ¼ cup rose hip seed oil

For dry skin:

- 1 tablespoon castor oil
- ¼ cup and 1 tablespoon rose hip seed oil
- 2 tablespoons avocado oil
- 2 tablespoons jojoba oil

For oily skin:

- 3 tablespoons castor oil
- ¼ cup and 3 tablespoons rose hip seed oil

DIRECTIONS

Combine the oils in a 4–8 ounce bottle and shake well.

HOW TO USE

Start by running a clean washcloth under hot water. Keep the water as hot as you can while still feeling comfortable—you don't want to burn yourself. Ring out the washcloth and place it over your face for about thirty seconds. Remove the washcloth, then drop about two teaspoons worth of oil cleanser into your palm, and then gently massage it onto your face and neck in a slow, circular motion. Continue to massage your skin for a minute or two. Run the washcloth under the hot water again, ring it out, and steam your face again for about ten seconds. Gently wipe the oil from your face, then repeat the steaming process two to three more times, or as many times as you feel you need to in order to remove all of the oil cleanser. Follow the cleanser with a toner, and if necessary, a moisturizer.

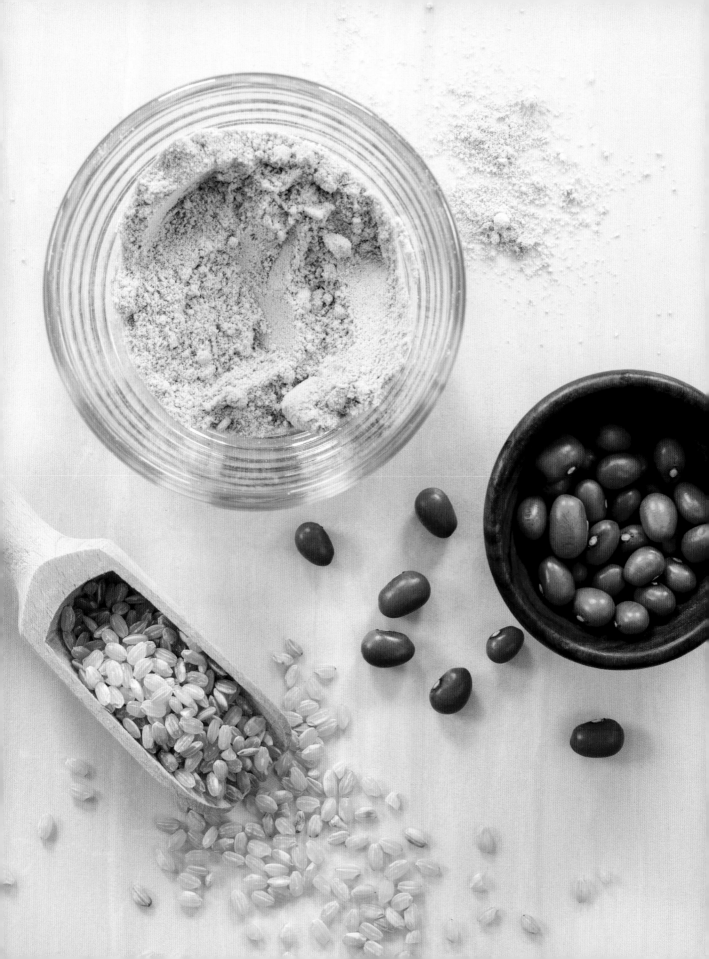

everyday recipe

WASHING GRAINS

Washing grains are incredibly simple to make and easy to use, making them a great first step into natural skincare. Washing grains work by gently exfoliating your skin while soaking up excess oil and scrubbing away dirt and grime. They are fabulous for all skin types, gentle enough to be used daily, and an excellent addition to any skin care routine. Even if you prefer using a different method for everyday cleansing, washing grains provide a great way to give your skin weekly or monthly exfoliation.

This recipe is one of the simplest, and most easy to use recipes that you'll find in this book. Adzuki bean powder is a gentle exfoliant, so this recipe can be used as an everyday cleanser. If you are using the oil cleansing method, or another daily facial care routine, this scrub can be used as an occasional treatment on a weekly or monthly basis.

The basic recipe works well for almost all skin types, and can easily be tailored to your specific needs.

- For dry and sensitive skin, try using kaolin clay and a soothing essential oil like roman chamomile or yarrow.

- For mature skin, you can use either kaolin or sea clay. Choose a balancing essential oil, such as rose or geranium.

- If you have oily or acne-prone skin, use sea clay and a 50/50 blend of niaouli and a soothing essential oil such as roman chamomile or yarrow.

TROUBLESHOOTING

Rosacea

Rosacea is a mysterious condition where the skin's blood vessels dilate, causing chronic redness of the skin. In some cases, it can be hard to distinguish between regular sensitive skin and rosacea. Rosacea is a case of blood vessels being overly sensitive, and while the exact cause is unknown, the condition seems to be more complex and deeply rooted than simply having a sensitive skin type. Some experts believe that certain cases of rosacea may be caused or aggravated by an imbalance in digestive bacteria. Other theories contend that rosacea is a genetic condition. If you find that your skin's redness doesn't improve with the use of a natural skin care routine or respond to anti-inflammatory ingredients, you may want to consult a dermatologist regarding the possibility of rosacea.

Washing Grains (continued)

INGREDIENTS

- ½ cup adzuki bean powder or rice bran powder or rice flour
- 3 tablespoons cosmetic clay
- 1 teaspoon baking soda
- 5–10 drops essential oil (optional)
- water or hydrosol, as needed

DIRECTIONS

Combine the powder and cosmetic clay in a small bowl and mix well. If you are adding essential oils, mix them with the baking soda in another bowl, then add the scented baking soda to the powder and clay mixture. Stir the powders well, making sure to break up any clumps that have formed in the powders. Transfer the mixture to a jar or powder sifter.

HOW TO USE

Wet your face and scoop about a teaspoon of the mixture into your palm. Add just enough water or hydrosol to form a smooth paste. Gently massage the paste onto your face in smooth, circular motions. Rinse with water and apply your toner and moisturizer as usual.

TROUBLESHOOTING

Acne

Recurring bouts of acne can be extremely frustrating. Commercial products often exacerbate the issue by over-drying or over-medicating skin that is already under distress. Rather than treating the symptoms, your best course of action for defeating acne is to root out its cause. Acne is most commonly caused by an overproduction of sebum, the skin's natural lubricant. Sebum can build up and clog pores, which leads to outbreaks, irritation, and spots. Often, getting your skin's oil-production balanced is enough to drastically reduce or even eliminate acne. This can be as easy as switching to a gentle, natural cleansing routine using Washing Grains or Cleansing Oils.

Another common cause for acne is bacterial or fungal infection. These can be treated by incorporating antibacterial and antifungal ingredients into your skin care routine. Try adding acne-fighting ingredients, like neem powder, niaouli essential oil, or karanja seed oil, to your recipes for Everyday Facial Cleanser, Cleansing Facial Oils, Moisturizing Facial Oils, or Facial Creams. Adding the Healing Facial Masque to your weekly or monthly routine can help too.

Other times, acne can be the result of something less obvious. Hormonal imbalances can play a big part, as can diet and undiagnosed allergies or sensitivities. If all else fails, consider consulting your doctor to have your thyroid and hormone levels evaluated. Or ask your doctor or nutritionist about going on an elimination or cleanse diet to identify any foods that might be stressing your skin.

everyday recipe

TONERS

The best all-natural toners, in my opinion, are hydrosols. Hydrosols are produced as byproducts of essential oils. The steam used to distill essential oils is collected and bottled as hydrosol, providing a beautiful water-based ingredient with a delicate aroma and mild herbal properties. Because hydrosols are so gentle, they can be used as-is for facial toners. You can use hydrosols alone, or blend them together to create something customized just for you.

INGREDIENTS

For normal skin:
- ¼ cup witch hazel hydrosol
- ¼ cup rose or rose geranium hydrosol

For sensitive skin:
- ¼ cup witch hazel hydrosol
- ¼ cup chamomile or yarrow hydrosol

For oily/acne prone skin:
- ¼ cup witch hazel hydrosol
- ¼ cup lavender or tea tree hydrosol

DIRECTIONS

Combine hydrosols in a 4 ounce bottle and shake well.

HOW TO USE

To use a hydrosol as a toner, simply open a bottle, moisten a cotton ball, and dab it generously onto your face. Toners should be used after cleansing your face and before applying a moisturizer.

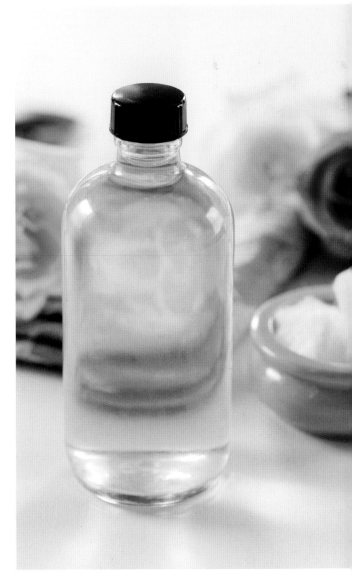

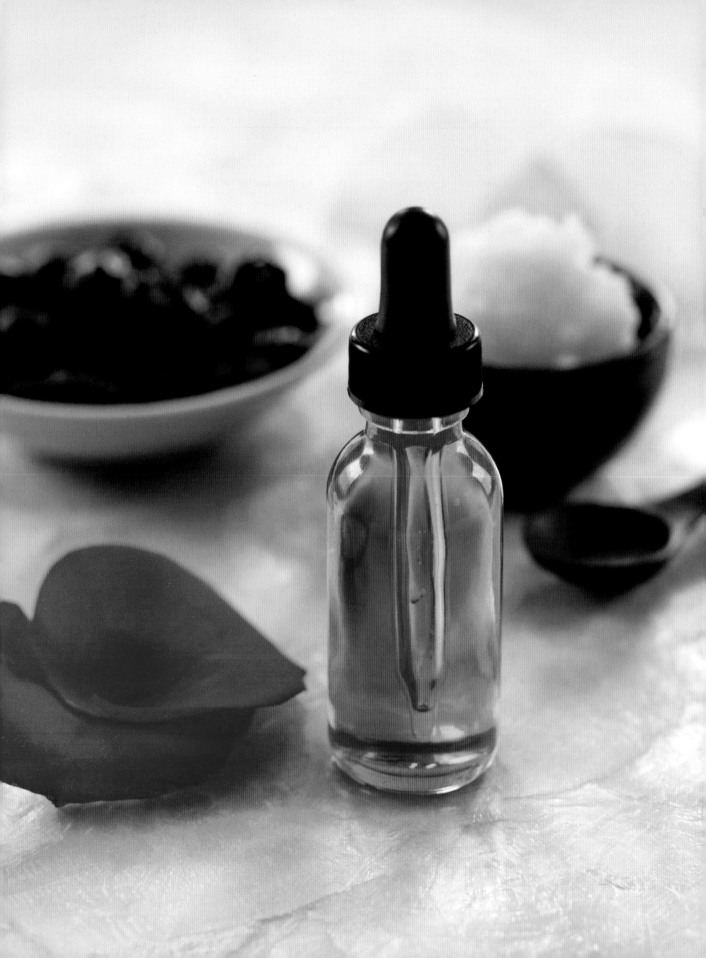

everyday recipe
MOISTURIZING FACIAL OILS

The easiest way to moisturize your skin naturally is by using moisturizing facial oils. Just a few drops of the right carrier oil can help keep your skin well-conditioned. Some carrier oils can even help repair damage, soothe irritation, and slow signs of aging. Best of all, moisturizing facial oils are easy to make and are shelf stable, meaning you can keep a batch in your bathroom for three to six months (depending on the oils you choose to use) without worrying about spoilage. Unlike creams and lotions diluted with water, wax, and other additives, moisturizing facial oils provide an intense punch of moisture. Think of them as moisturizing serums for your skin.

If you are used to using creams and lotions, facial oils will take a little getting used to. The oils won't absorb immediately, and the slightly greasy feeling on your skin might be unpleasant at first. Make sure to go light on the oil, especially when you are just getting started, and give your skin some time to adjust to the new routine. It usually takes only a few drops to moisturize your face and neck for an entire day.

You can beef up your facial oil blend by incorporating essential oils or specialty carrier oils. Try swapping out one of the basic carrier oils with something more exotic, such as tamanu or pomegranate seed oil. Essential oils should be well-diluted so they don't irritate your skin. Skin-safe essential oils can be added at a rate of 6–12 drops per ounce of facial oil.

	MATURE SKIN	ACNE-PRONE OR COMBINATION SKIN	SENSITIVE SKIN
Preferred Carrier Oils	Argan Oil Evening Primrose Oil Pomegranate Oil	Karanja Seed Oil Perilla seed Oil	Oat Oil Raspberry Seed Oil Tamanu Oil
Optional Add-Ons	Geranium Essential Oil Helichrysum Essential Oil Rose Essential Oil	Acne-Prone: Niaouli Essential Oil Combination: Geranium Essential Oil	Chamomile Essential Oil Yarrow Essential Oil

Moisturizing Facial Oils (continued)

> ## INGREDIENTS <

For normal skin:

- 1 tablespoon rose hip seed oil
- 1 tablespoon apricot kernal oil or watermelon seed oil

For dry or sensitive skin:

- 1 tablespoon rose hip seed oil
- 1½ teaspoons jojoba oil
- 1½ teaspoons avocado oil

For oily or acne prone skin:

- 1 tablespoon rose hip seed oil
- 1 tablespoon organic virgin coconut oil

> ## DIRECTIONS <

Combine oils in a 1-ounce bottle and shake well.

> ## HOW TO USE <

After cleansing and toning your face, apply a few drops of oil to your bare hands. Gently massage the oil onto your face in a gentle, circular motion. The oil will take some time to absorb. If you find that the oil is interfering with makeup application, or if it isn't soaking into your skin quickly enough, try using fewer drops, or applying the moisturizer before bed instead of in the morning.

TROUBLESHOOTING

Eczema

Like acne, the most important thing to determine when battling eczema is the cause. Eczema can be caused or aggravated by a variety of sensitivities, both internal and external. First, try eliminating all artificial dyes and fragrances from your routine. Ditch everything from scented laundry detergents to perfumes and chemical air fresheners, then give your skin a couple of weeks to adjust to the change.

If you still aren't seeing any improvement, it's possible that the eczema is a result of a food allergy or sensitivity. Uncovering a food sensitivity can be tricky. The best way to solve this mystery is to go on an elimination diet. By eliminating the most common foods related to eczema then slowly reintroducing them, you can figure out exactly what foods are causing the problem. The most common food

sensitivities related to eczema are gluten, dairy, eggs, and citrus. Consult your doctor or allergist to plan an elimination diet, then monitor your skin closely as the foods are reintroduced..

In some cases, eczema can persist even after chemical and food sensitivities are ruled out. If you can't eliminate the eczema, the next best thing is to find a skincare routine that helps alleviate its symptoms. An all-natural routine is often best for eczema. Focus on using ingredients that are suitable for sensitive and dry skin. Anti-inflammatory oils or butters like pomegranate oil and murumuru butter can be used as-is to moisturize, or they can be incorporated into simple recipes like facial creams or body butters.

everyday recipe
FACIAL CREAMS

Creams and lotions are made using a simple process called *emulsion*. This process encapsulates water within a microscopic net of oils and wax. The result is a wet, fluffy cloud of moisturizing goop that we tend to go gaga for. The drawback to creams and lotions is that the moisturizing oils and butters they contain have been diluted with water, wax, and additives. Commercial creams and lotions often contain powerful preservatives, thickening agents, alcohol, chemical dyes, and fragrances. It's easy to see how the very products that are meant to nourish our skin can cause serious irritation.

Thankfully, fresh creams can be made at home in small batches with relative ease. Really, it isn't much more complicated than whipping up a homemade salad dressing. One thing to keep in mind when making fresh facial creams, however, is that like homemade salad dressings, they have a short shelf life. Because cream contains water, it is very fragile, and prone to bacterial growth. It's important to store your homemade creams in the refrigerator between uses, and to avoid handling them directly whenever you can. Plan on tossing your current batch and whipping up a fresh one every week to keep ahead of spoilage.

The following basic facial cream recipe can be customized by swapping out all or a portion of the rose hip seed oil with a different carrier oil. The addition of essential oils is optional. Choose an essential oil tailored to your skin type, or pick one that works well on all types of skin, like rose or geranium. The water can also be swapped out for a hydrosol suited to your skin type.

	MATURE SKIN	ACNE-PRONE SKIN	SENSITIVE SKIN
Preferred Carrier Oils	Argan Oil Evening Primrose Oil Pomegranate Oil	Karanja Seed Oil Neem Oil Perilla Seed Oil	Oat Oil Raspberry Seed Oil Tamanu Oil
Optional Add-Ons	Geranium Essential Oil Helichrysum Essential Oil Rose Essential Oil	Geranium Essential Oil Niaouli Essential Oil	Chamomile Essential Oil Yarrow Essential Oil
Replace water with	Geranium Hydrosol Rose Hydrosol	Lavender Hydrosol Witch Hazel Hydrosol	Chamomile Hydrosol Yarrow Hydrosol

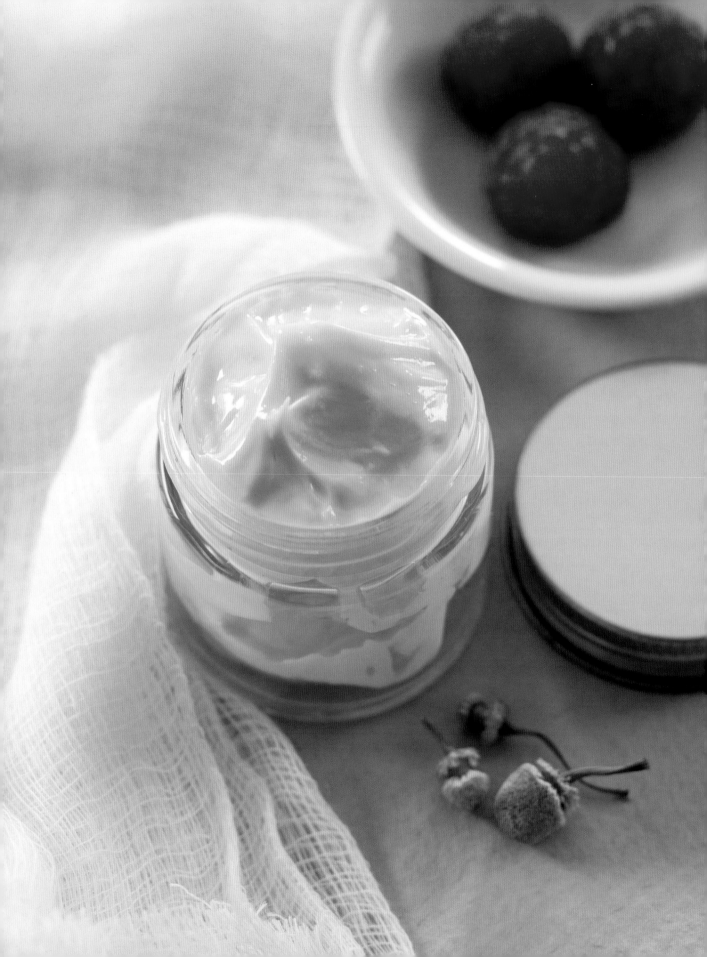

Facial Creams (continued)

INGREDIENTS

- ¼ teaspoon borax
- 2 tablespoons distilled water or hydrosol
- 1 teaspoon beeswax or candelilla pellets
- ¼ teaspoon lecithin
- 2½ teaspoons rose hip seed oil
- 2½ teaspoons virgin coconut oil
- 10 drops essential oil (optional)

TROUBLESHOOTING

Candida and Other Fungal Infections

Fungal skin infections, like candida, can cause redness, acne, itchiness, and inflammation. Often, these conditions arise as a result of an imbalance, not only in your skin's pH, but also in your body's digestive system. In addition to treating fungal skin problems topically, taking a probiotic supplement, or introducing safe fermented foods into your diet can help a lot. Reducing the amount of sugar and alcohol in your diet can also contribute to a speedy recovery. As far as skin care goes, be extra careful to make sure that all of your products are fresh, and that the tools you are using (washcloths, cotton cosmetic pads, etc.) are clean and sterile. Antifungal ingredients, like neem oil and niaouli essential oil can be incorporated into your routine for an extra boost of fungus-fighting power. It can also be helpful to consult a doctor or naturopathic physician to get help with these kinds of infections, especially if you are dealing with something persistent or severe.

Natural Beauty Tip

Fresh creams and lotions don't contain the heavy-duty preservatives that make store-bought lotions shelf stable. Handmade lotions and creams should be used within one week, or stored in the refrigerator for up to three weeks.

DIRECTIONS

Mix the borax into the water or hydrosol and stir until the borax has completely dissolved. Gently warm the borax mixture. This can be done at a low heat on the stove top or in 15 second bursts in the microwave. Melt the beeswax and mix it with the lecithin and rose hip seed oil. (Ideally, the borax mixture and the wax mixture should both be hot when they are mixed together.) Begin whisking the oil and wax mixture and slowly pour the borax mixture into it. Whisk the mixture continuously for at least five minutes. (This is much easier when using an electric hand mixer.) The mixture should thicken as it cools, resulting in a fluffy cream. Stir the essential oils (if using) into the mixture last and then transfer to a 2-ounce jar. To see photos of this process, check out page 16.

HOW TO USE

After you've applied your toner, apply a few dabs of cream to freshly cleansed skin. Gently massage the cream into your skin in a slow, circular motion. Homemade creams will feel heavier than the commercial creams you might be used to. Give the cream some extra time to absorb. If you find it to be too greasy, try using a little bit less cream on your next try, or consider switching to a moisturizing facial oil instead.

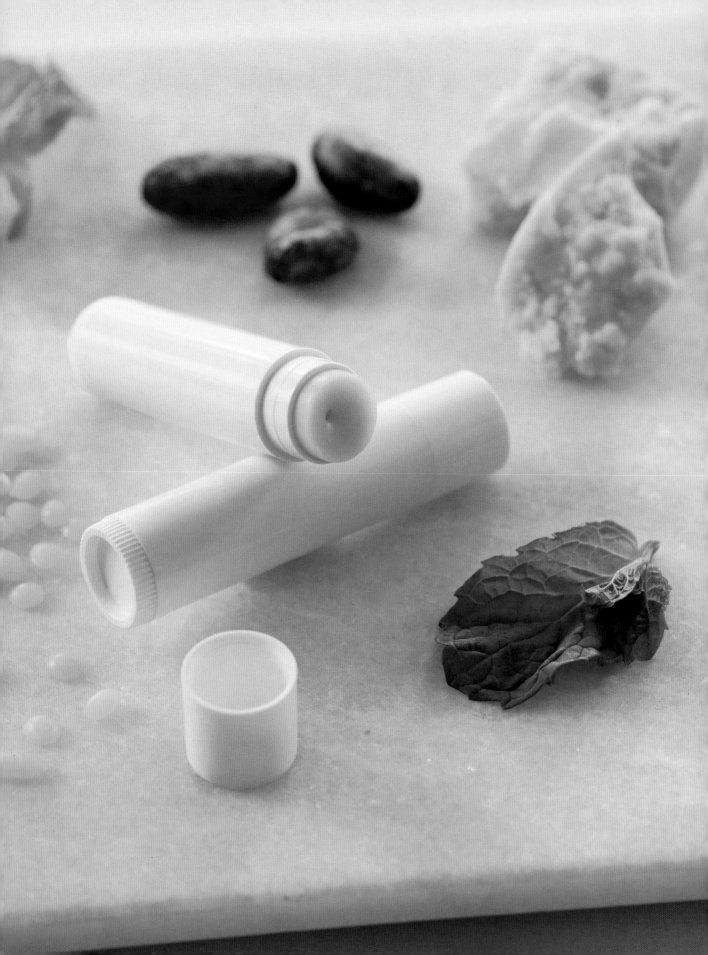

everyday recipe

LIP BALMS

Making your own lip balm is simple, inexpensive, and surprisingly fun. A small batch makes multiple balms, enough to keep you well stocked for an entire season, or enough to share with family and friends. Since handmade lip balms don't contain water, they are fairly stable. You can expect a batch of lip balms to last from six months to a year. While commercial lip balms are sometimes made with icky ingredients, such as mineral oil and artificial fragrances, homemade lip balms can be made with the best, most lip-nourishing ingredients around. Once you start making your own balms, you'll wonder how you ever had eyes for Chapstick.

> INGREDIENTS <

For basic lip balm (fills about 15 lip balm tubes):

- ¼ cup beeswax pellets
- 2 tablespoons shea butter or cocoa butter
- 1 tablespoon jojoba oil
- 1 tablespoon avocado oil
- ½ teaspoon peppermint essential oil (optional)
- 1 teaspoon liquid lecithin

For vegan lip balm (fills about 12 lip balm tubes):

- 2 tablespoons and 1 teaspoon candelilla wax
- 2 tablespoons shea butter or cocoa butter
- 1 tablespoon jojoba oil
- 1 tablespoon avocado oil
- ½ teaspoon peppermint essential oil (optional)
- 1 teaspoon liquid lecithin

> DIRECTIONS <

Melt the wax and the shea or cocoa butter in a double boiler, or in the microwave. If you are using the microwave, melt the ingredients in short, 30 second bursts, stirring in between each one. Add the jojoba and avocado oils and stir well. Add the peppermint essential oil (if using) and the liquid lecithin, and stir again, then carefully pour the mixture into your lip balm tubes. Allow the lip balms to cool and harden completely before moving or using them.

> HOW TO USE <

Apply liberally to your lips anytime they are feeling chapped or dry.

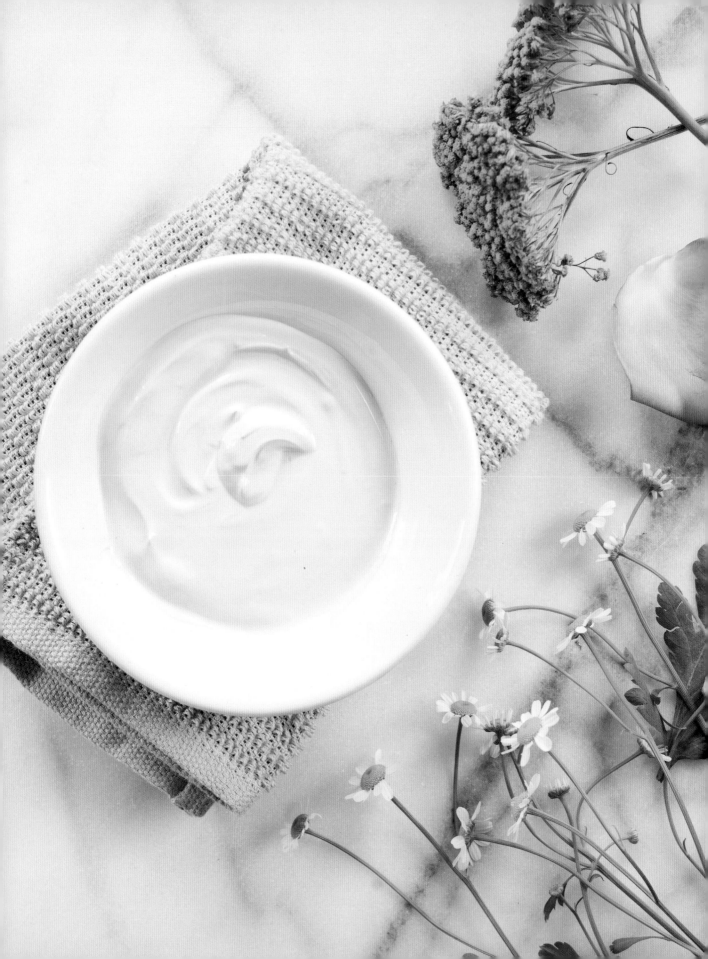

specialty recipe

DEEP CLEANSING MASQUE

While washing grains and facial oils are great for everyday care, it's awfully nice to pamper your skin once in a while with a fresh masque. Not only will your skin benefit from a deep cleansing, your mood is sure to benefit from taking the occasional break to relax and care for your body. This basic clay masque helps to draw out excess oil, toxins, and other impurities that can build up in your skin.

This masque is great for all skin types, but you can replace the cosmetic clay with something stronger if you have oily or acne-prone skin. Try using French green clay or illite clay in place of the kaolin clay. Just be careful not to let your skin become overly dried by these powerful clays. If you are using a gentle clay, such as kaolin clay or rose clay, you can use this kind of masque as often as you like. Some even enjoy using a gentle facial masque as part of their daily routine. Masques that include strong clays, like French green or illite clay, should be used only once a week—even on oily skin.

To customize this masque, replace the water with a hydrosol suited to your skin type. Including a few drops of essential oil can boost the benefit even further.

	MATURE SKIN	ACNE-PRONE OR COMBINATION SKIN	SENSITIVE SKIN
Optional Add-Ons	Geranium Essential Oil Helichrysum Essential Oil Rose Essential Oil	Niaouli Essential Oil	Chamomile Essential Oil Yarrow Essential Oil
Replace water with	Rose Hydrosol or Rose Geranium Hydrosol	Lavender Hydrosol or Witch Hazel Hydrosol	Chamomile Hydrosol or Yarrow Hydrosol

⟩ INGREDIENTS ⟨

- 2 tablespoons kaolin clay
- 1–2 tablespoons water or hydrosol
- 1–3 drops essential oil (optional)

⟩ DIRECTIONS ⟨

Mix the clay with just enough water or hydrosol to form a smooth paste. If using, mix in the essential oil and stir well.

⟩ HOW TO USE ⟨

Apply the masque to your face and neck by spreading it over the skin in slow, circular motions. Allow it to dry for about ten minutes before rinsing. It may not harden completely before it is time to rinse it off. Follow with the toner and moisturizer of your choice. This recipe should be used right away, but any unused portion can be stored in a sealed container in the refrigerator for up to one week.

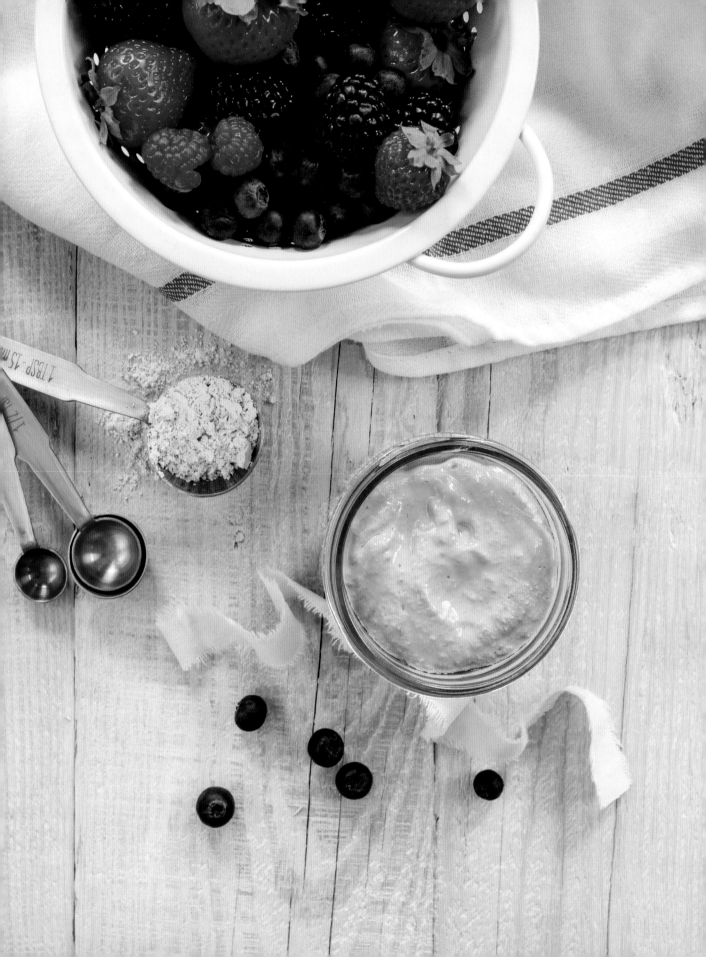

specialty recipe

ALPHA HYDROXY FACIAL

Did you know that the goodies in your fruit bowl contain gentle acids that are perfect for scrubbing away dull, dead skin? These mild acids, called alpha-hydroxy acids, have a talent for loosening dead skin cells, increasing the effectiveness of exfoliation, thus brightening skin. Yogurt is another excellent ingredient for gentle exfoliation as it contains natural lactic acid. Lactic acids work similarly to alpha-hydroxy acids, lifting dull layers of skin without irritation.

Whipping up a fresh alpha hydroxy acid treatment every once in a while is an easy way to keep your skin looking its best. I recommend indulging in this kind of treatment on a weekly or monthly basis. Of course, it doesn't hurt to throw one together whenever the mood strikes. It's best to use organic fruits and dairy for this recipe whenever possible. To create a vegan version, simply omit the yogurt, and add a little bit of water or extra fruit instead.

INGREDIENTS

- ½ cup organic berries
- 2 tablespoons organic plain yogurt
- 2 tablespoons kaolin clay
- water or hydrosol, as needed

DIRECTIONS

Combine the berries, yogurt, and kaolin clay in a blender and puree until smooth. If you don't have a blender, simply mash the berries with the other ingredients to form a paste. If the mixture is too thick to spread easily, add a little bit of water or hydrosol to loosen it up.

HOW TO USE

Apply the mixture liberally to your face and neck. Allow the mixture to dry for about ten minutes, then use your fingers to gently massage the mixture into your skin using slow, circular motions. Rinse with tepid water, then follow with a toner and moisturizer. This recipe should be used right away, but can be stored in a sealed container in the refrigerator for up to three days.

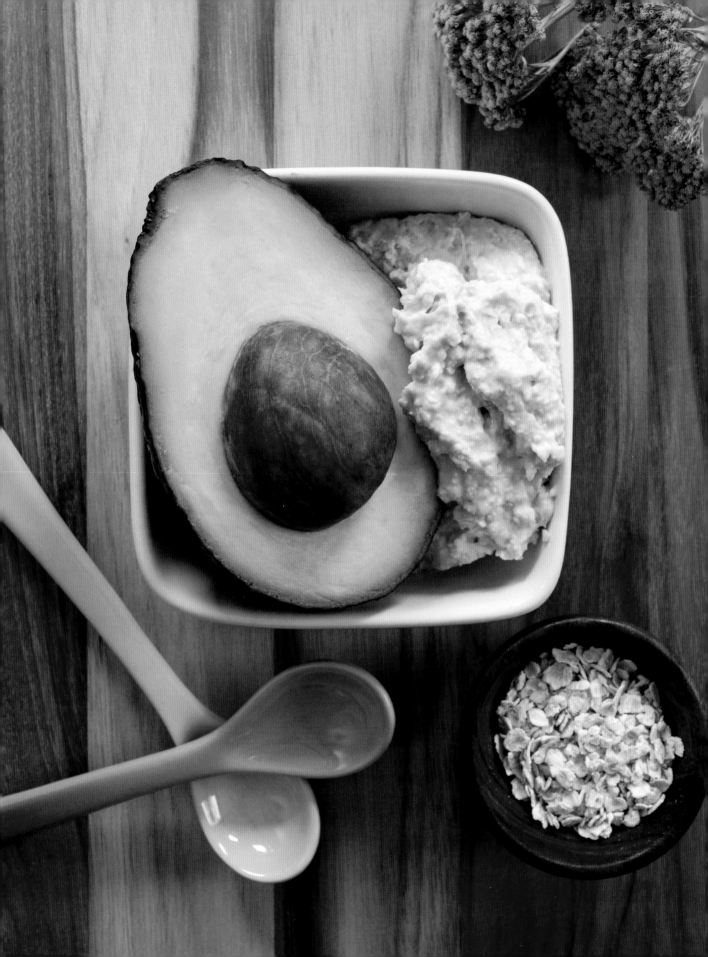

specialty recipe

SOOTHING OAT & AVOCADO MASQUE

This masque starts off with a simple emulsion of oil and hydrosol, then adds in a few of my favorite skin soothing ingredients. Soothing oats, creamy avocado, and nourishing yogurt soothe and condition the skin while the anti-inflammatory essential oils work to reduce redness and irritation. After twenty minutes with this masque on, even the grumpiest skin will be more content. This masque is gentle enough to be used on a daily basis, but it's rich texture and indulgent ingredients make it better suited for occasional use.

INGREDIENTS

- 1 tablespoon facial cream
  (recipe on page 51)
- 2 tablespoons whole oats or oat flour
- 1 tablespoon fresh avocado, mashed
  or pureed
- 2 tablespoons organic plain yogurt
- 10 drops yarrow or chamomile essential oil

DIRECTIONS

Combine the ingredients in a blender or food processor and pulse until combined. Add extra yogurt if the mixture is too thick to blend easily.

HOW TO USE

Apply the mixture liberally to your face and neck. Allow the masque to sit on your skin for about twenty minutes, then gently wipe it away with a warm damp cloth. This masque will not harden as it dries. This recipe should be used fresh, but leftovers can be stored in the fridge for up to three days.

PROFESSIONAL HELP

SPF

When it comes to protecting your skin from sun damage, it's best to stick to professionally manufactured products. While there are many natural ingredients that contain elements that can help stop sun damage, it's impossible to know exactly how much sun protection a homemade recipe will offer. Sun Protection Factor (SPF) values are determined using sophisticated lab testing. In fact, it's against FDA regulations to market a product as containing SPF value without those tests having been conducted. That being said, not all sun care products are created equal. For the healthiest choice possible, make a habit of reading the back of the bottle and scrutinizing ingredients. Seek out natural products that don't contain paraben preservatives, synthetic dyes, and artificial fragrances. The Environmental Working Group offers a consumer guide to shopping for sunscreens (at *www.ewg.org*) that includes detailed ingredient information and safety ratings. Whatever brand you choose, be sure to apply sunscreen daily. Unprotected exposure can lead to premature aging, skin damage, and even cancer.

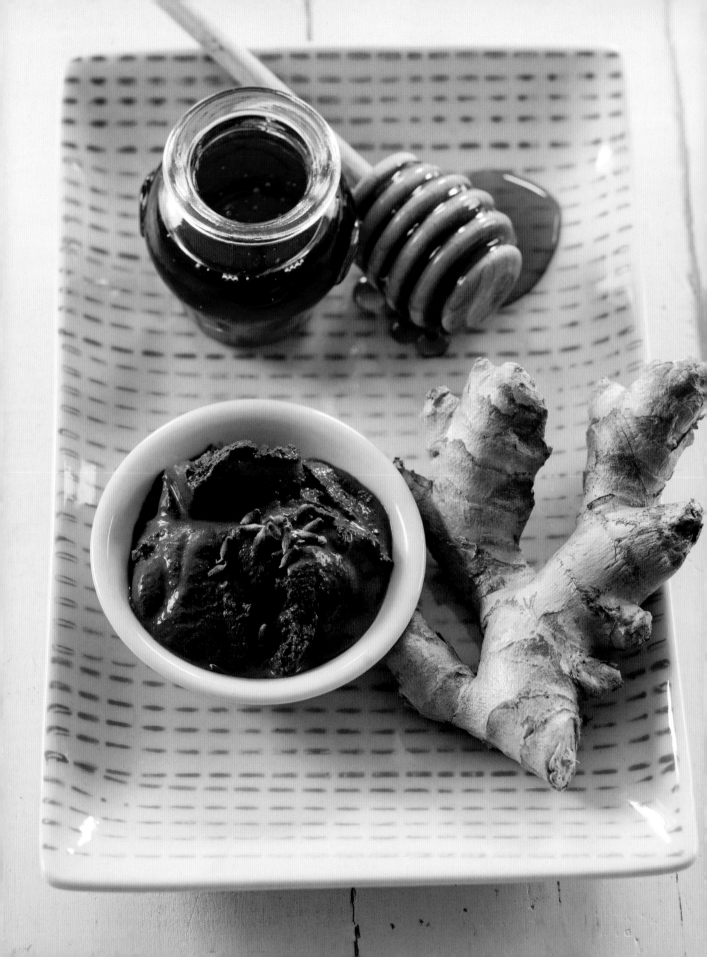

specialty recipe

HEALING FACIAL MASQUE

Acne, irritation, and even some forms of rosacea can be caused by the presence of unwanted bacteria or fungus in the skin. Nature has provided us with excellent ingredients that can help ward off these kinds of skin care villains. The following masque can be used on a weekly or monthly basis to keep bacteria and fungus at bay. Sea clay is a good choice for most skin types, but if your skin is particularly dry or sensitive, use kaolin instead.

INGREDIENTS

- 2 tablespoons sea clay or kaolin clay
- 1 tablespoon ginger powder
- 1 teaspoon honey
- 1 – 2 tablespoons lavender or witch hazel hydrosol
- 1 teaspoon neem oil, karanja seed oil, or perilla seed oil
- 6 drops niaouli essential oil

HOW TO USE

Apply the masque to your face and neck. Allow the masque to dry for about ten minutes before rinsing. It may not harden completely before it is time to rinse. Follow with a toner and moisturizer. This recipe should be used fresh, but leftovers can be stored in the fridge for up to three days.

DIRECTIONS

Combine the sea or kaolin clay and ginger powder in a small bowl. Add the honey and hydrosol or witch hazel, then mix into a paste. Add the oil and essential oils, and stir well. The mixture should form a smooth paste. If it is too dry, add a little more hydrosol, as needed.

ask a
NATURAL BEAUTY
EXPERT

Q: What kind of DIY recipes do you enjoy making the most? Do you tend to favor everyday recipes or are you more inclined to create specialty treatments?

A: I love making everyday recipes, but I think the fresh ingredients in specialty recipes is where natural ingredients really come into their own, because like fresh food, fresh beauty ingredients contain active ingredients the cosmetic companies would kill for.

Cybele Masterman, blahblahmagazine.com.au

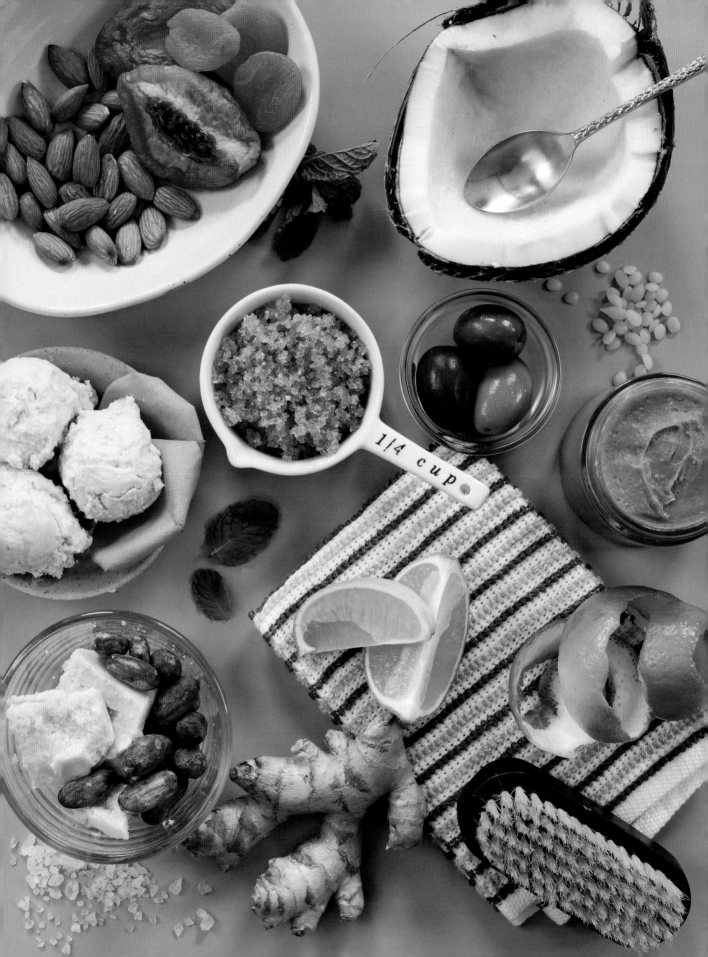

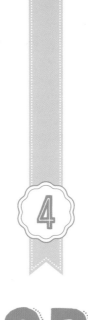

BODY

We tend to focus on our face and hair when it comes to beauty, but the rest of your body deserves a healthy routine too. When you consider the surface area of your body that is exposed to harsh detergents and synthetic toxins on a daily basis, it makes perfect sense to make detoxifying your bodycare routine a priority. Luckily, switching up your bodycare routine can be as simple as swapping out commercial body washes and lotions with all-natural soaps, handmade body butters, and simple scrubs. Crafting your own homemade deodorant is an extra step that you can take to totally free yourself from commercial products.

Commercially produced body washes and detergent soap bars are packed with toxic additives and can be extremely drying and irritating. Switching to all-natural bar soap is the first, and simplest step in changing your body care routine. This small change can reduce redness, inflammation, and dryness. Natural soaps are made from moisturizing oils and butters while commercial soap bars are often nothing more than a solid block of detergent. Where body washes and detergent soap bars » strip the skin of beneficial oils, natural soaps actually help supplement them.

Making your own bar soap can be a rewarding project, but it's okay to save yourself time and effort by purchasing natural bar soap from a local artisan or natural food store. Look for soaps that are cold-processed, fragrance-free, and made with pure vegetable oils. These are the best bars to use in hand-milled recipes, and they are the gentlest on your skin when used as-is. Castile soap is the easiest to find, and is often available in grocery stores in the natural living section.

Moisturizing your skin provides another excellent opportunity for improvement. Commercial lotions and body butters are often bulked up with water and alcohol—not to mention synthetic preservatives, additives, and fragrances. Like junk food, these types of lotions provide pleasure, but very little actual nourishment. While they might feel great on your

dry skin, the moisture they provide is often fleeting. Handmade body butters and body oils, on the other hand, offer intensive conditioning and the benefit of ingredients packed with vitamins, antioxidants, and essential fatty acids.

You'll find that handmade body butters and body oils are usually thicker and greasier than commercial lotions. This can take a little getting used to, as the pure oils and natural butters need extra time to be absorbed. Another thing you'll notice is that their effect is far more longlasting, so you won't need to apply them as often as you would commercial lotions. In fact, most people only need to apply body butter or body oil once a day to ensure perfectly moisturized skin.

WHAT TO EXPECT

For the most part, switching to a natural body care routine is very straightforward. The skin on our arms, legs, and torso isn't usually as sensitive as our faces and scalps, so you shouldn't experience the kind of intense adjustment period that you might with changing your facial or hair care routine. While giving up the rich foaming lathers and perfumed scents that come along with commercial body products might take a little getting used to, your skin won't mind at all. In fact, you may see a reduction in redness, dryness, and sensitivity right away.

---

ask a
NATURAL BEAUTY EXPERT

Q: Do you have any advice for maintaining a successful natural beauty routine?

A: My best tip for keeping up your routine is to use your planner and stick to it. Tuesday is a deep conditioning night for my hair. Every Tuesday and Friday I exfoliate, and I cleanse and moisturize on a daily basis. After a few weeks it just feels wrong not to stick to my schedule.

Twila Dawn Willis, The Herb Bar
theherbbar.com

everyday recipe

HAND-MILLED SOAP BARS

Cleansing your skin should be a simple affair, and it doesn't get much more simple than good old-fashioned soap. While there is absolutely no shame in buying a pre-made bar of natural soap, many people find soap making to be fun and rewarding hobby. Hand milling is a great technique for beginning soap makers as it offers an opportunity for creativity without the exacting calculations needed for making soap entirely from scratch.

When purchasing soap base to work with, look for soaps made with pure saponified oils. Castile bars from Vermont Soap, Austin Natural Soap, or Castile Rebatch Base from Bramble Berry all work really well. Avoid any bars or bases that contain salt, as the soap won't melt as easily.

If you are feeling adventurous, this basic hand-milled soap recipe can be easily customized by including some of the following add-ins.

	ALL SKIN TYPES	OILY / ACNE-PRONE SKIN	DRY / SENSITIVE SKIN
Carrier Oils or Butters	Apricot Kernel Oil Shea Butter	Neem Oil Organic Virgin Coconut Oil	Avocado Oil Cocoa Butter
Clays	Kaolin Clay	French Green Clay Sea Clay	None (see recipe)
Exfoliants	Adzuki Bean Powder Almond Meal Ground Coffee Rolled Oats		
Essential Oils	Peppermint Essential Oil Rose Essential Oil	Lavender Essential Oil Niaouli Essential Oil	Chamomile Essential Oil Yarrow Essential Oil
Liquids	Beer Green Tea Water	Honey	Aloe Vera Gel Chamomile Tea

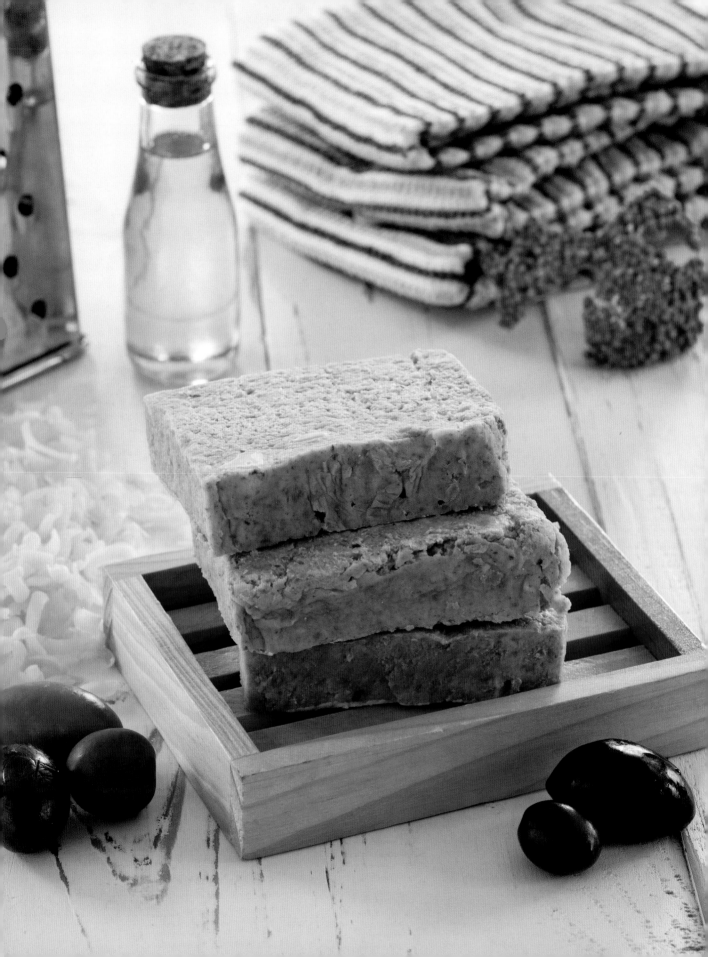

Hand-Milled Soap Bars (continued)

INGREDIENTS

- ☐ 1 pound natural castile bar soap, shredded
- ☐ ½ cup plus two tablespoons water
- ☐ 2 tablespoons carrier oil, honey, or vegetable butter
- ☐ 2 tablespoons clay (omit for dry skin) or exfoliant
- ☐ 2 teaspoons essential oil (optional)

DIRECTIONS

Combine the shredded soap and ½ cup water in a double boiler or crock pot set to low. Heat the mixture, stirring often, until fully melted. Combine the clays and/or exfoliants with the remaining two tablespoons of water, then add them to the melted soap. Finally, stir in any additives you're using, such as essential oil, honey, or carrier oil. Transfer the soap to a silicone mold or a wooden mold lined with wax paper. Allow the soap to cool and set until it is hard enough to handle. This could take up to three days. When the soap has hardened, gently remove it from the mold and slice it into four bars. Set the bars on a rack to dry for one to three weeks. The bars are ready to use when they are fully hardened and dry. For photos of this process, check out page 18.

HOW TO USE

These bars should lather pretty well, so you can enjoy them as-is or rub them into a pouf or washcloth for extra bubbles. Lather the bubbles all over, from your shoulders to toes, then rinse.

PROFESSIONAL HELP

Bar Soap

While soap making can be a fun and rewarding hobby, this is an area where I heartily encourage you to cheat. Natural and even handmade soaps are readily available. They can be found online, in many grocery stores, and at farmers' markets. When shopping for soap, look for bars that are all-natural, cold-processed, and when possible, handmade. 100% pure castile soap is easy to find, as Dr. Bronner's is sold in most grocery and natural food stores. I prefer unscented soap, but you can find natural soap scented with a wide variety of essential oils. If you are shopping for scented soap just be sure to check the label. If you see fragrance listed as an ingredient that means it contains synthetic perfume—a notoriously irritating and possibly harmful substance.

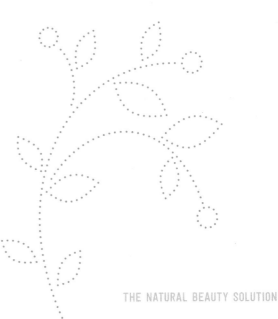

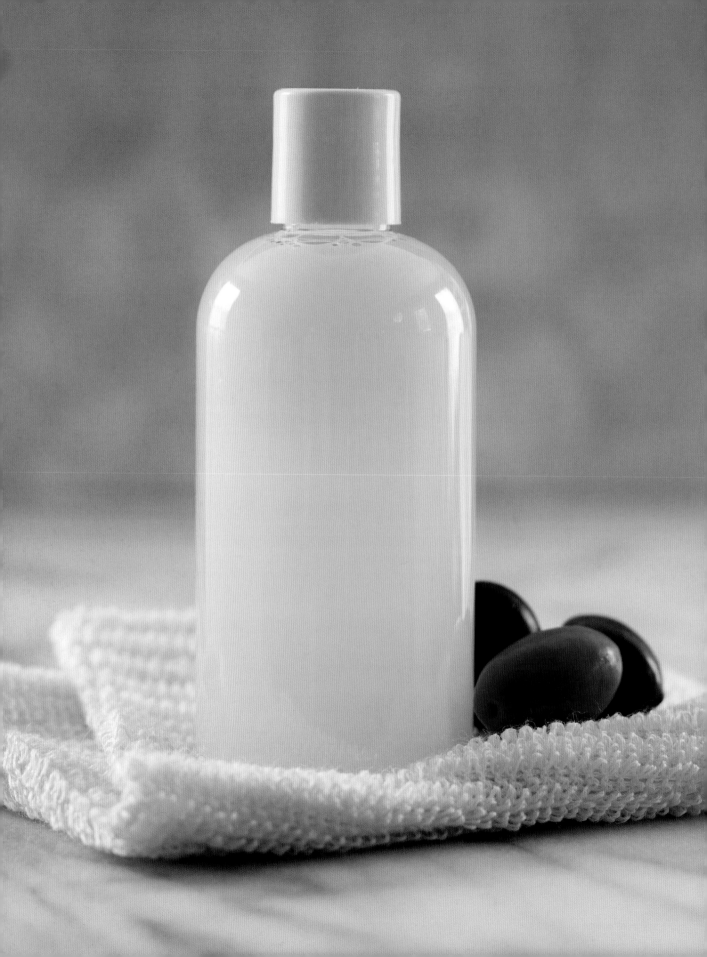

everyday recipe

CASTILE BODY WASH

This all-natural body wash is a far cry from what you'll find on the shelves of a beauty shop, but it's also much more gentle. The concentrated liquid soap can be diluted with either aloe vera gel, hydrosol, or just plain water—depending on how involved you'd like to get while customizing the recipe. Essential oil can also be added to give the body wash a pleasant scent or add customized skin care properties.

	ALL SKIN TYPES	OILY / ACNE-PRONE SKIN	DRY / SENSITIVE SKIN
Gels or Hydrosols	Aloe Vera Gel Neroli Hydrosol Rose Hydrosol Rose Geranium Hydrosol	Lavender Hydrosol Witch Hazel Hydrosol	Aloe Vera Gel Chamomile Hydrosol Yarrow Hydrosol
Essential Oils	Peppermint Essential Oil Rose Essential Oil	Niaouli Essential Oil Lavender Essential Oil	Chamomile Essential Oil Yarrow Essential Oil

> INGREDIENTS <

- 12 ounces water, aloe vera gel, or hydrosol
- 4 ounces liquid castile soap
- 1 teaspoon essential oil (optional)

> DIRECTIONS <

Combine all ingredients in a 16-ounce bottle and shake slowly to combine.

> HOW TO USE <

This body wash will have a very thin texture, and will lather a little less than the commercial body washes you may be used to. Scrunch it up into a moistened bath sponge, poof, or washcloth to get the most bubbles possible.

TROUBLESHOOTING

Persistently Dry Skin

If your skin insists on being dry even after you switch to an all-natural routine, you may need to take extra steps. The first thing I'd recommend doing is switching to the Castile Body Wash, and diluting it with an extra 4 to 8 ounces of water. Next, try to moisturize head to toe with body oil or body butter at least twice every day. Here are a few more tips to help beat dry skin naturally:

- Drink plenty of water. Hydration is essential to happy skin.
- Include healthy fats in your diet from foods like salmon, avocado, and virgin coconut oil.
- Avoid bathing or showering in extremely hot water. The extra heat can dry your skin.

If your dry skin continues or escalates, consider seeing a doctor or dermatologist. Chronically dry skin can be a symptom of stress, undiagnosed allergies, or underlying health problems.

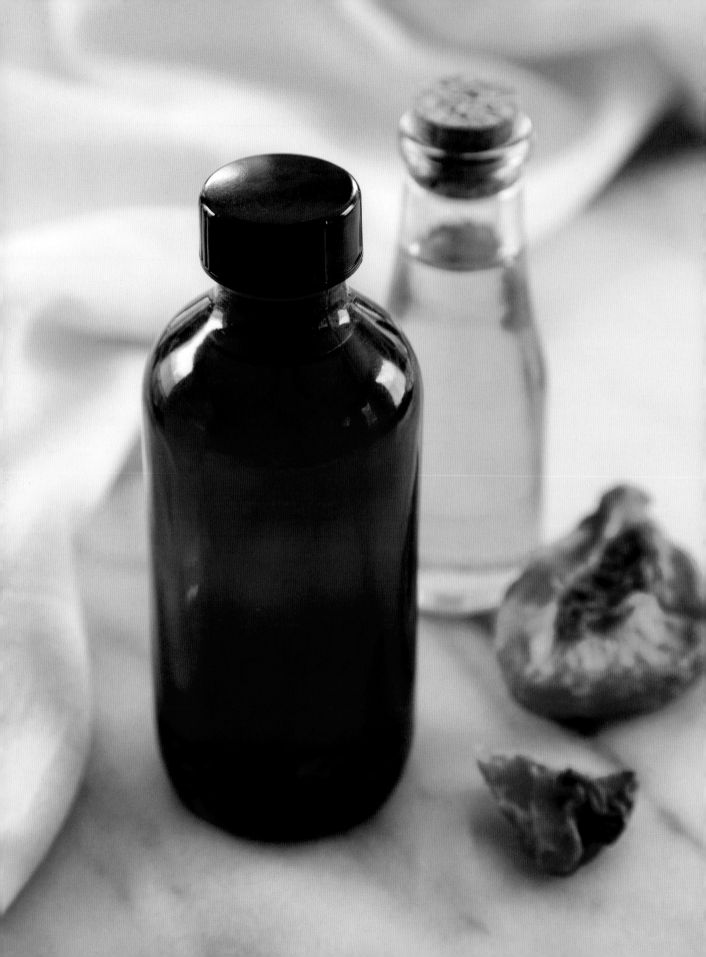

everyday recipe

BODY OIL

It doesn't get much simpler than body oil when it comes to moisturizing your skin. The right oil blend will be light, easily absorbed, and nourishing and will leave your skin healthy and happy. Body oils are great for post-shower moisturizing and can be applied head to toe quickly and easily, keeping your skin well conditioned for the rest of the day. As an added bonus, body oils can be used for massage.

Essential oils can be added to enhance the scent of your body oil, and even provide some aromatherapy benefits. Here are a few suggestions for how you can add therapeutic scent to your body oil:

- A soothing essential oil, like roman chamomile or yarrow would be great for sensitive skin.
- Rose or neroli essential oils can be included to give your body oil a lovely feminine scent.
- If you'd like to give your body oil a cooling, stimulating feeling, try adding peppermint essential oil.

INGREDIENTS

- ½ cup watermelon seed oil or apricot kernel oil
- ¼ cup organic virgin coconut oil
- ¼ cup avocado oil
- ½ teaspoon essential oil (optional)

DIRECTIONS

Combine ingredients in an eight ounce bottle and shake well.

HOW TO USE

I like using my body oil right after I step out of the shower. Pour a few teaspoons of oil into the palm of your hand, then massage it onto your arms, legs, and torso. It will take a few minutes for the oil to absorb into your skin. Make sure it has soaked in before getting dressed. to avoid getting any on your clothes.

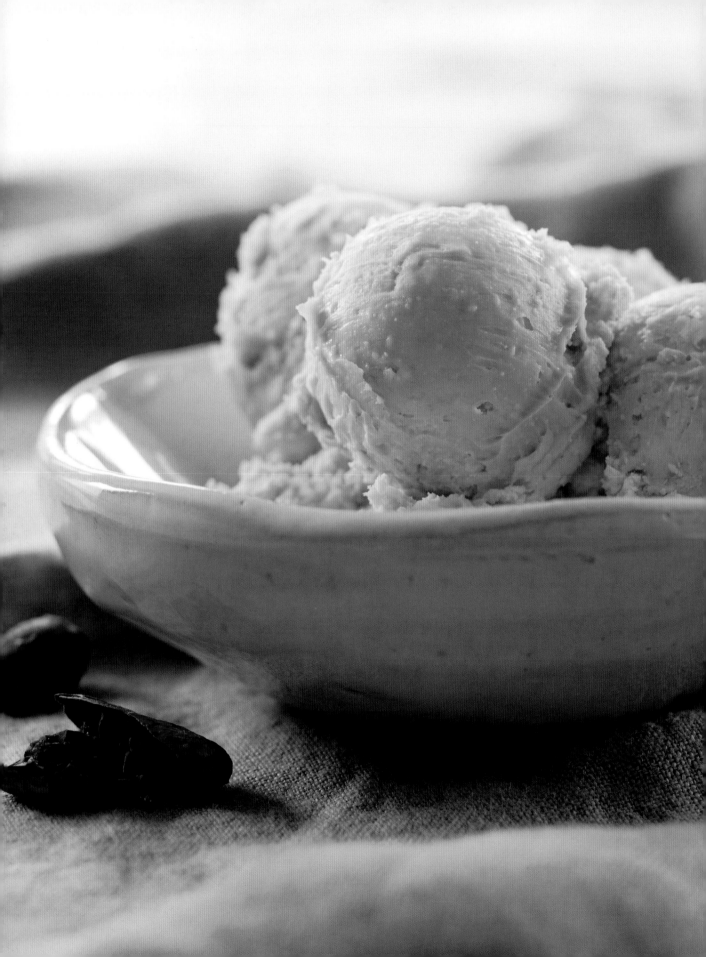

everyday recipe

BODY BUTTER

Body butters are made from a simple mixture of vegetable butter, carrier oil, and natural wax. The result is a thick balm that provides intense moisture—perfect for dry spots such as your elbows, knees, and feet. If you are prone to dry skin, try using a body butter all over for lasting protection. Body butters are fairly easy to make. The ingredients are melted together, then cooled—solidifying as they reach room temperature. Body butters can be left to cool as-is or whipped as they cool to give them a lighter, fluffier texture.

This recipe can be left unscented, or you can add a little bit of rose or neroli essential oil to make it extra wonderful.

Unhappy Hands

When I lived in the Northeast, my hands would become extremely dry during the winter. Brutal cold, dry air, and constant changes in temperature made keeping my hands happy and healthy a serious challenge. If you are facing a similar dilemma, or if there are other factors that make your hands extra susceptible to dry skin there are a few extra steps you can take to battle dryness.

- **Embrace balms and body butters**. Creams and lotions feel lovely on dry skin, but they are bulked up with water. Balms and body butters pack a more intensive punch, being made from straight butters, oils, and waxes.

- **Wear gloves.** An easy overnight treatment for extremely dry hands uses cotton gloves to seal in moisture. Before going to bed, apply a thick layer of balm or body butter to your hands, then cover them with cotton gloves. Your skin will absorb the oils while you sleep, softening and moisturizing your hands.

- **Stay hydrated.** It's important to keep drinking plenty of water during cold weather. Even though you may not feel it, dry air from heaters and winter weather can dry you right out. If you are too chilly to drink cold water, try heating it up! Drinking hot water during the winter is a great way to stay hydrated and comfortable.

Body Butter (continued)

INGREDIENTS

- ½ cup shea butter
- ¼ cup apricot kernel oil
  or watermelon seed oil
- 1 tablespoon beeswax pellets
- 1 teaspoon essential oil (optional)

DIRECTIONS

Combine the butter, oil, and wax in a double boiler or a crockpot set to low. Heat until the ingredients are fully melted. Remove the mixture from the heat, and let sit for a few moments. Stir in the essential oil (if using). The butter can be transferred to a 6-ounce jar at this point and cooled until firm, or you can whip the butter to give it a fluffy texture.

A WHIPPED VARIATION

To create a whipped butter, whisk the butter continuously until it cools and thickens. This may take several minutes, so using an electric hand mixer will help make the task easier. If your butter seems especially stubborn about setting up, try nesting your mixing bowl in a larger bowl packed with ice. Be careful not to splash any water into the body butter. When the mixture has thickened up transfer the whipped butter to a jar and refrigerate it until it sets into a hard butter. Keep in mind while choosing a container for your body butter that the mixture will increase in volume after being whipped. Try packaging the whipped butter in an eight to ten ounce jar.

HOW TO USE

Body Butter can be applied liberally to your arms, legs, and torso. It's even great for your hands and feet. Massage the butter into your skin in a circular motion. It is greasier than lotion and store-bought butters made with water, so it will take some extra time to absorb.

everyday recipe

BODY LOTION

A little more complex than body butter, crafting handmade body lotion may take a little bit of practice. Lotions involve a special process called *emulsion* that binds the water and oil phases together. The final product is lighter and thinner than body butter or body oil, but still much thicker and heavier than the store-bought lotions that you might be used to. Commercial lotions often include fillers, extra binding agents, and synthetic additives to give them their extremely light and fast-drying textures.

While they might feel lovely on the skin, ingredients like silicone, alcohol, and mineral oil don't offer much in the way of actual conditioning. This explains why you might find yourself applying your favorite store-bought lotion again and again throughout the day. Homemade lotion, on the other hand is packed with moisturizing ingredients that will leave your skin moisturized and protected far more effectively.

Body lotion can be left unscented or enhanced with the essential oil of your choice. Try adding peppermint essential oil to give your lotion a cooling effect or add a floral essential oil like rose, neroli, or geranium to give it an attractive aroma.

Natural Beauty Tip
Fresh creams and lotions don't contain the heavy-duty preservatives that make store-bought lotions shelf stable. Handmade lotions and creams should be used within one week, or stored in the refrigerator for up to three weeks. Make sure to label the lotion so it won't end up on anyone's sandwich.

TROUBLESHOOTING

Tackling Emulsion

Getting a lotion or a cream just right can sometimes be a frustrating endeavor. It's not at all unusual for beginners it see their emulsions break down and separate, even after measuring properly and carefully following directions. In this way, lotion making is a little bit like learning to bake. The formula behind each recipe is crucial, but so is the technique used to put it all together. When working on emulsions, keep the following tips in mind:

- The oil and water phases should be as close in temperature as possible when mixed.
- Add the water phase to the oil phase in a steady stream, whisking continuously.
- The cream or lotion must be whisked for at least ten minutes in order to stabilize.

Body Lotion (continued)

> INGREDIENTS <

- 2 tablespoons avocado oil
- 2 tablespoons apricot kernel oil or watermelon seed oil
- 2 tablespoons shea butter or cocoa butter
- 1 tablespoon beeswax pellets
- 1 teaspoon lecithin
- ¼ cup and 2 tablespoons water or hydrosol
- 1 teaspoon borax
- ½ teaspoon essential oil (optional)

> DIRECTIONS <

For the oil phase, combine the oils, butter, wax, and lecithin in a double boiler and heat until the ingredients have fully melted together. The water phase is next. Combine the water or hydrosol with the borax in a second pan. Heat the water phase until it becomes hot, but try not to let it boil. Remove both mixtures from the heat, then begin whisking the oil phase. While whisking vigorously, carefully pour the water phase into the oil phase in a slow, steady stream. Whisk continuously as the lotion cools and thickens. Continue whisking for at least five minutes. Stir in any essential oils you are using last. Then transfer to an 8-ounce bottle with a pump or a disc cap. To see photos of this process, check out page 16.

> HOW TO USE <

This moisturizing body lotion can be applied liberally from your shoulders to your toes. Massage it into your skin, giving it a little extra time to absorb than you would a store-bought lotion.

PERSONAL STORIES

How I Broke My Fragrance Addiction

As a child I was a classic tom-boy. I preferred dinosaurs and astronauts to pink ponies and ballerinas. When I discovered the world of girly bath and body products as a teenager it was a total surprise. I was instantly in love, and started collecting scented lotions, body scrubs, and bath bombs with gusto. I even invested in a bottle of expensive French perfume. Meanwhile I was struggling with itchy red skin, breakouts, and acne. It didn't occur to me at the time that these things could be connected, but years later I realized that all of those fun flirty fragrances were driving my skin crazy. I gave them up for the sake of clear skin, but it hurt a little.

Nowadays I still love a yummy scented body product, but I keep the sources natural. Neroli hydrosol makes an excellent body spray. I keep a small spray bottle on hand to spritz my hair and skin whenever I'm missing the feeling of perfume. Naturally aromatic ingredients like virgin coconut oil or rose essential oil let me add feminine scents to other homemade recipes like body butters, body oils, and bath products.

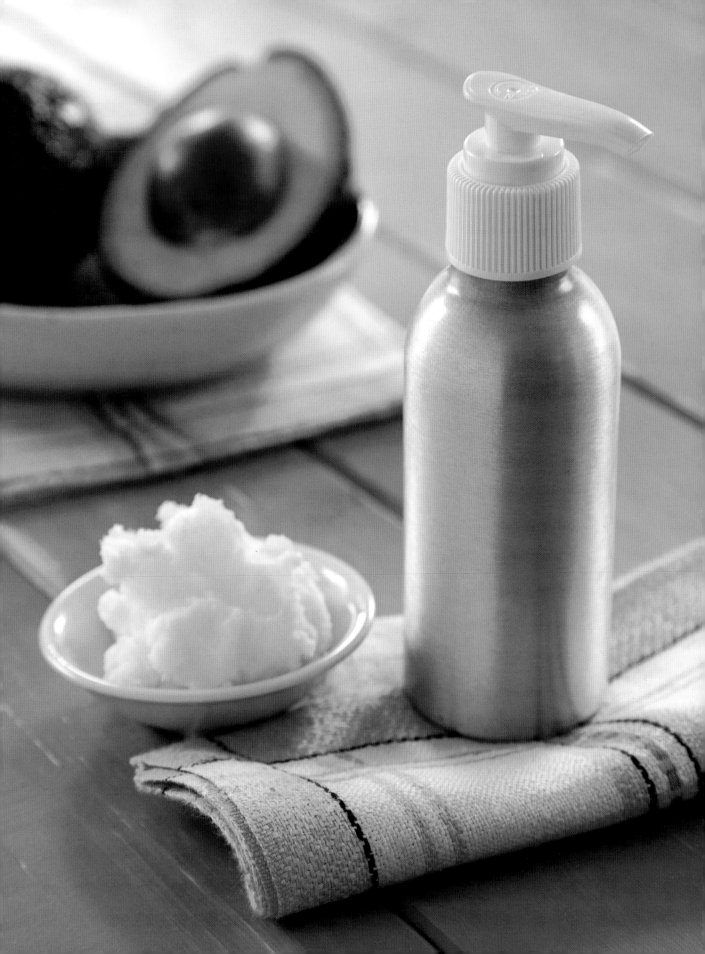

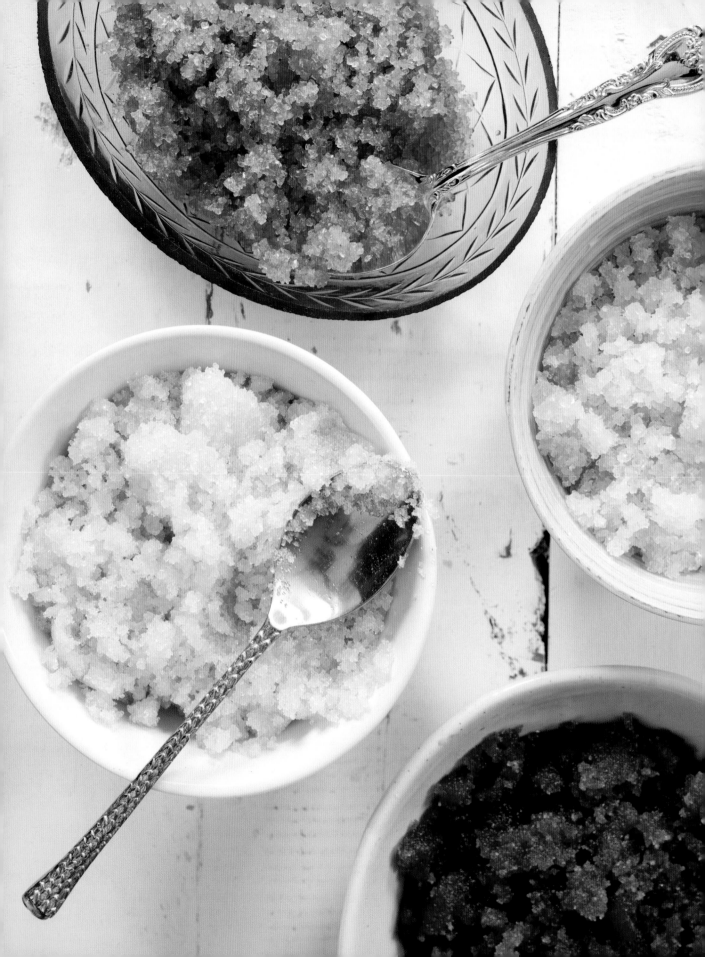

everyday recipe

SUGAR AND SALT SCRUBS

Even the healthiest skin can get a little rough around the edges as cells die and are replaced. One surefire way to keep your skin smooth and soft is to exfoliate regularly. Salt and sugar scrubs are easy to make and can be created quickly and affordably at home. In fact, scrubs require only two ingredients. This might make you wonder why boutiques and beauty shops charge so much for something so painfully simple. Commercial scrubs are usually quite simple to start with, using cheap oils and even cheaper salt or sugar. Most are loaded with synthetic dyes and fragrances but dressed up in a fancy package that likely costs more to produce than the scrub itself!

If you are wondering whether to use salt or sugar in your scrub, consider this: Salt provides extra benefits by way of natural mineral content. Sugar exfoliates just as well, but doesn't sting when exposed to cuts or scrapes. This makes salt a great choice for foot scrubs and all-over scrubs, while sugar is a better choice for scrubs that accompany shaving routines or for those with highly sensitive skin.

If you'd like to jazz up your basic scrub, try adding an essential oil. Peppermint will lend a cool, tingly feeling. Rose or neroli essential oil will add a flirty floral aroma.

INGREDIENTS

- ½ cup fine sugar or sea salt
- 2–4 tablespoons apricot kernel oil or watermelon seed oil
- ½ teaspoon essential oil (optional)

DIRECTIONS

Add the salt or sugar to a small mixing bowl. Begin adding the oil, and keep adding it until the mixture reaches a consistency that you like. Some people prefer a drier scrub, while others like them to be a little on the loose side. Just go with whichever you prefer. Stir in any essential oil you are using last.

An assortment of scrubs made with (from top) turbinado sugar, sea salt, organic sugar, and brown sugar

HOW TO USE

Moisten the skin on your arms, legs, torso, hands, or feet, then apply a small scoop of scrub into the palm of your hand. Rub the scrub onto your skin in a slow, circular motion until it crumbles away completely. Repeat until you've scrubbed everywhere you need exfoliation. One batch of scrub should be enough to exfoliate your whole body, from shoulders to toes. These scrubs are great for body care, but would be too rough for the delicate skin of your neck and face. This recipe makes enough for one or two full body scrubs. To avoid contaminating your scrub, scoop the portion you plan to use right away into a paper or plastic container that you can bring with you into the bathroom. The remaining scrub can be stored as-is in a sealed jar for up to one month.

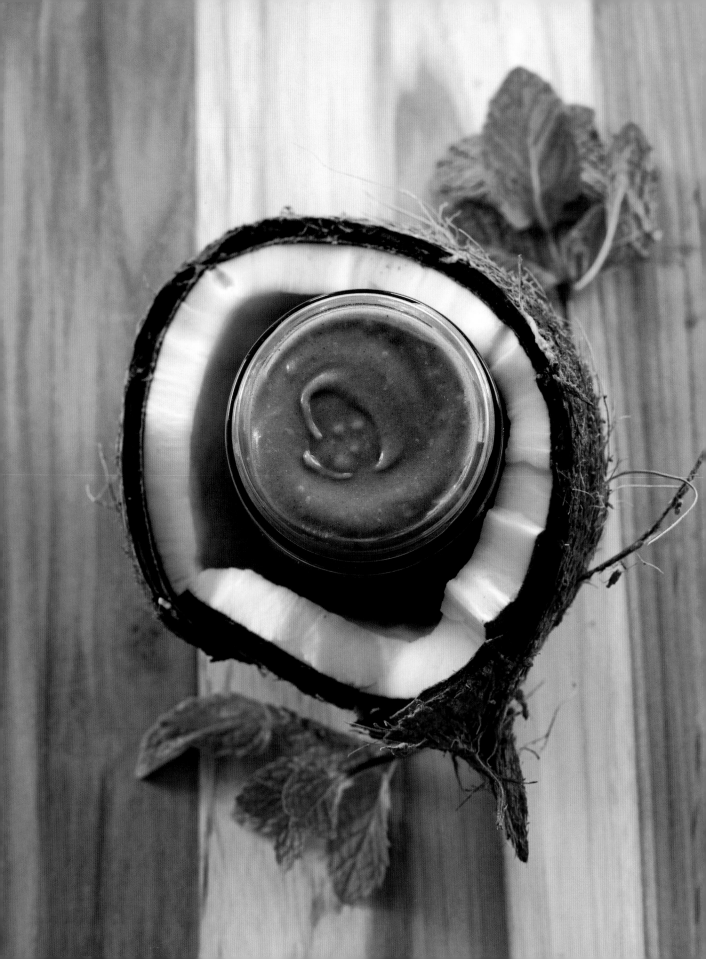

everyday recipe

DEODORANT

Commercial deodorants can contain some pretty scary stuff; aluminum, parabens, and synthetic fragrances just to name a few. Unfortunately, these are often the same ingredients that make commercial deodorants and antiperspirants so effective. Homemade deodorant is probably the single most challenging aspect of an entirely natural and handmade skin care routine—simply because personal preference and expectations can vary a lot.

Keep in mind that unlike antiperspirant, homemade deodorant won't stop you from sweating. What it can do is help to keep your underarm bouquet from becoming overpowering. There are a few special ingredients in this recipe that may be a little harder to find than other everyday recipes in this book. The oils, butters, and essential oils used in this recipe work by battling the bacterias that cause underarms to smell funky. Clay and baking soda are included to help absorb scent and moisture. Additional essential oils should be added according to your personal preference. Some of my favorites for ladies' deodorants are neroli, rose, and ylang ylang. Fir, juniper, and sandalwood provide more masculine scents. Mandarin, basil, and spearmint are great for unisex blends.

TROUBLESHOOTING

Irritated Underarms

Some people find that homemade deodorants irritate the sensitive skin under their arms. If this happens to you, it could be due to the presence of baking soda or the type of essential oil in the recipe. Baking soda can sometimes unbalance the skin's pH, and certain people may discover that their skin has a sensitivity to some essential oils. Try making a batch without the baking soda or without the essential oil. A more simple formula might work better for your particular skin type.

Deodorant (continued)

> INGREDIENTS <

- ☐ 6 tablespoons organic virgin coconut oil
- ☐ 1 tablespoon karanja seed oil
- ☐ 2 tablespoons beeswax pellets
- ☐ ¼ cup baking soda
- ☐ 2 tablespoons bentonite clay
- ☐ 2 tablespoons cornstarch
- ☐ ½ teaspoon niaouli essential oil
- ☐ ½ teaspoon additional essential oil (optional)

> DIRECTIONS <

Combine the coconut oil, karanja seed oil, and wax in a double boiler or crockpot set to low and heat until fully melted. In a separate mixing bowl, whisk the baking soda, bentonite clay, and cornstarch together. Remove the oil and wax mixture from the heat, wait a few moments for the mixture to cool off slightly, then stir in any essential oils you are using. Slowly combine the powder and oil and wax mixtures, whisking continuously to avoid clumps. Carefully pour the mixture into two 4-ounce jars. Allow the mixture to cool and set completely before use.

> HOW TO USE <

This recipe will produce a semi-solid balm, best stored in a small lidded jar or airtight plastic container. To use, scoop a small dab of the balm out of the jar with your fingers, then rub it into your underarms. The deodorant can be used once in the morning, or throughout the day as necessary.

Natural Beauty Tip

Homemade deodorant is made with all-natural ingredients which could potentially stain or darken clothing. I haven't personally had a problem with deodorant staining my clothes, but I have heard of it happening to other people. My advice would be to proceed with caution while wearing anything bright white or particularly delicate. For example, you might not want to try this recipe out in your wedding dress—just in case!

specialty recipe
WARMING MASSAGE OIL

When discussing body care, I would be remiss to leave out a special oil for massage. While you can massage with pretty much any carrier oil, this blend includes special ingredients that can help encourage blood flow by warming and stimulating the skin. When combined with a strong pair of hands this warming massage oil makes short work of stiff joints and sore muscles. The scent of the essential oils in this recipe can be quite strong. If you prefer a milder aroma, try cutting the amount of essential oil used in half or omitting it from the recipe altogether.

INGREDIENTS

- ½ cup watermelon seed oil
  or apricot kernel oil
- up to 24 drops ginger essential oil
- up to 48 drops black pepper essential oil

DIRECTIONS

Combine ingredients in a 4 ounce bottle and shake well.

HOW TO USE

Pour about a teaspoon of massage oil into the palm of your hand, then rub your hands together to warm the oil. Place your palms onto the area you plan to massage, then rub your palms gently over the skin. Reapply the oil as needed during your massage.

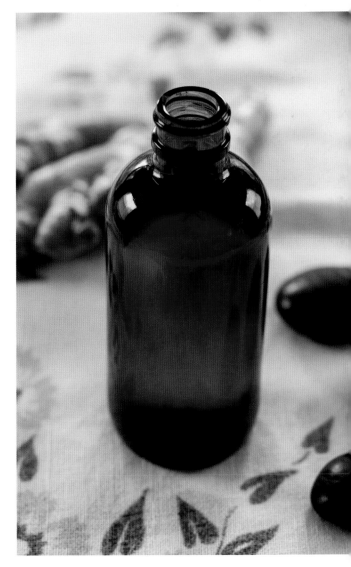

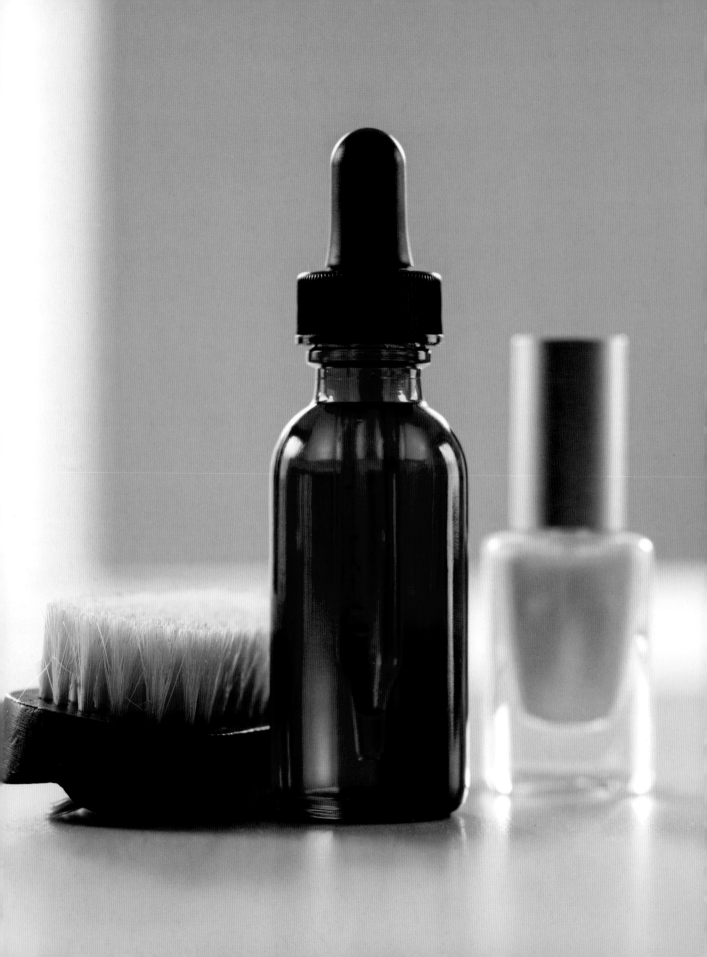

specialty recipe

CUTICLE OIL

Taking good care of your hands and nails is an important, but often overlooked part of an overall beauty routine. Besides keeping your hands well-moisturized and safe from harsh detergents and extreme temperatures, it helps to keep your fingernails nicely manicured. Your cuticles, the thin layers of skin at the base of your fingernails, can be damaged easily by everyday abuse. When they are kept neat and well moisturized they are less likely to be cracked, snagged, or torn. Keeping the skin intact reduces the risk of infection, inhibits the growth of calluses, and can discourage the buildup of dead skin. This simple cuticle oil is excellent for softening hard cuticles before and after a manicure. After tackling your cuticles, your nails can be filed and buffed for a totally natural look that compliments both women and men.

INGREDIENTS

- 2 tablespoons avocado oil
- 18 drops niaouli essential oil

DIRECTIONS

Combine the avocado and essential oils in a 1-ounce dropper bottle and shake well.

HOW TO USE

Before starting your manicure, it's good practice to sterilize any of your reusable tools. Drop your nail clippers, cuticle scissors, and stainless steel cuticle stick into boiling water for a few minutes before use to kill any germs that may be lurking on them. Use a heat-proof pair of tongs to remove the sterilized equipment, and be careful not to burn yourself.

Apply one drop of cuticle oil to the base of each fingernail. Rub the oil into the cuticle, then let them sit for two to three minutes. Use a cuticle stick to push the cuticles down from the fingernail, then use cuticle scissors or clippers to carefully trim away any excess dead skin. Be careful not to trim into the healthy cuticle or the skin around your fingernails. If you see redness or blood (or if you are experiencing any pain) you have gone too far! Finish by applying another drop of oil to each fingernail and massaging it in.

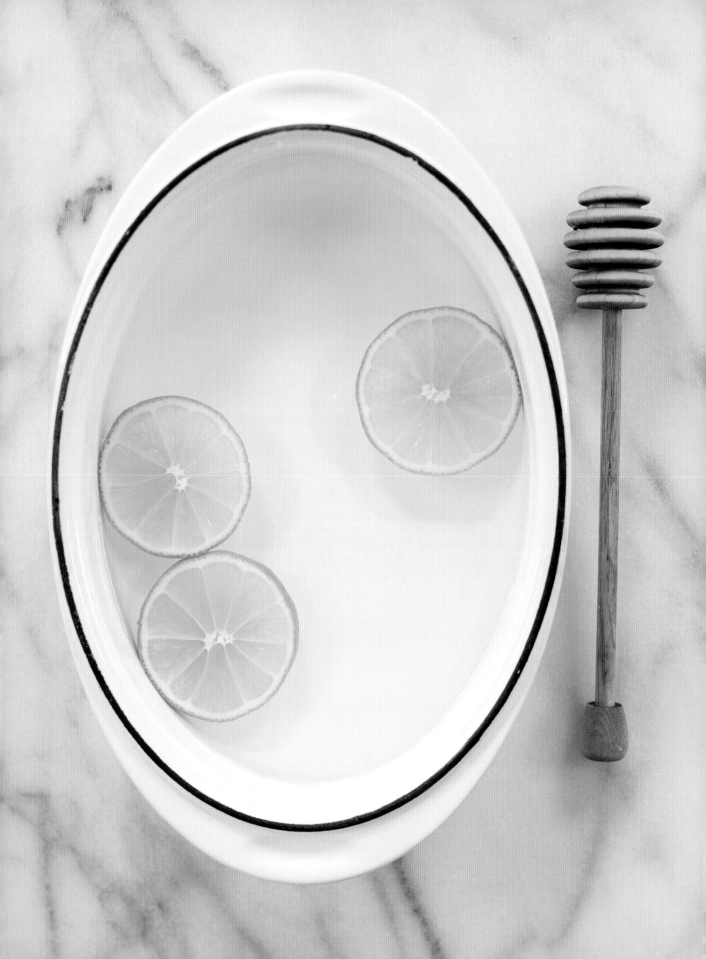

specialty recipe

PEDICURE SOAK

This easy-to-brew foot soak combines natural ingredients that can help soothe and disinfect even the most disheveled pair of feet. Epsom salt is included to encourage circulation and relieve soreness and stiffness. Honey, lime, and niaouli essential oil help discourage bacteria that causes itching and stinky feet.

INGREDIENTS

- 1 cup epsom salt
- 1 gallon hot water
- 1 teaspoon niaouli essential oil
- 1 tablespoon honey
- 1 fresh lime, juiced

DIRECTIONS

Dissolve the epsom salt into the hot water. In a small bowl, mix the essential oil with the honey. Add a little of the hot salt water to the mixing bowl and stir until the honey has dissolved. Add the lime juice, then pour the mixture into a foot bath along with the remaining hot salt water.

HOW TO USE

Soak your feet in the hot mixture for at least fifteen minutes or until the water cools to room temperature. Pat dry, then follow with a scrub and pedicure.

PROFESSIONAL HELP

Natural Nail Care

The nail salon can be a scary place. Most salons don't select their products with much scrutiny, so you will find your hands and feet bathing in synthetic dyes, irritating fragrances, and toxic chemicals. For example, did you know that acetone is a nerve toxin? Stop for a moment and consider just how many really important nerve endings live in your hands and feet. Yikes! Luckily, natural nail care is a growing trend, making it easier to find salons that cater to clients with a natural lifestyle. I'm not particularly talented at DIY manicures and pedicures, so I choose to seek out natural nail care salons about once a season for a major overhaul on my hands and feet. If you love the ritual of mani-pedi pampering as much as I do, I suggest doing the same.

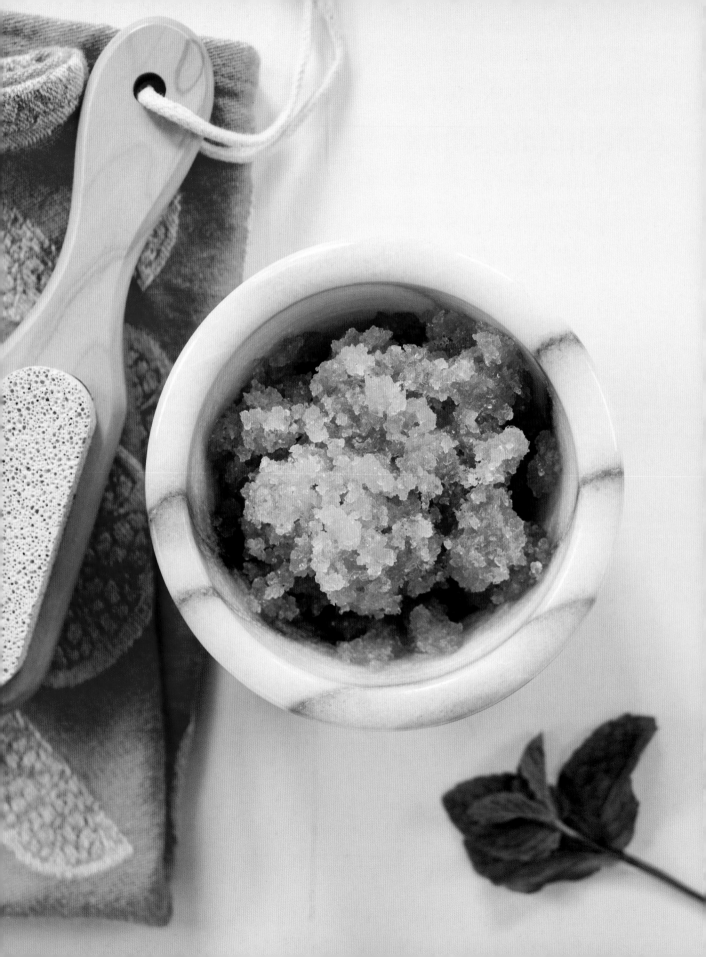

specialty recipe
PEDICURE SCRUB

Follow your foot soak with this extra-exfoliating pedicure scrub, which includes naturally abrasive ingredients and an extra boost of antibacterial essential oils to keep your feet smelling spiffy after the pedicure is over. Moisturizing avocado oil helps condition your feet, leaving them smooth, soft, and happy. This recipe makes enough scrub to thoroughly polish one pair of feet. I suggest using the whole batch at once. If you'd like to keep some for later, save the portion you'd like to keep in a small jar, and scoop the portion you plan to use immediately into a small plastic or paper container. The reserved scrub will last as-is for up to one month.

⟩ INGREDIENTS ⟨

- ½ cup fine sea salt
- 3 tablespoons avocado oil
- 1 tablespoon karanja seed oil or neem oil
- ¼ teaspoon peppermint essential oil
- ¼ teaspoon niaouli essential oil

⟩ DIRECTIONS ⟨

Combine the ingredients in a small mixing bowl and stir well.

⟩ HOW TO USE ⟨

Rub the mixture vigorously onto freshly soaked feet. Massage the scrub into the skin in a slow circular motion until the scrub crumbles away. Rinse with water, then pat dry. Take extra care after using this scrub as your feet may be slippery!

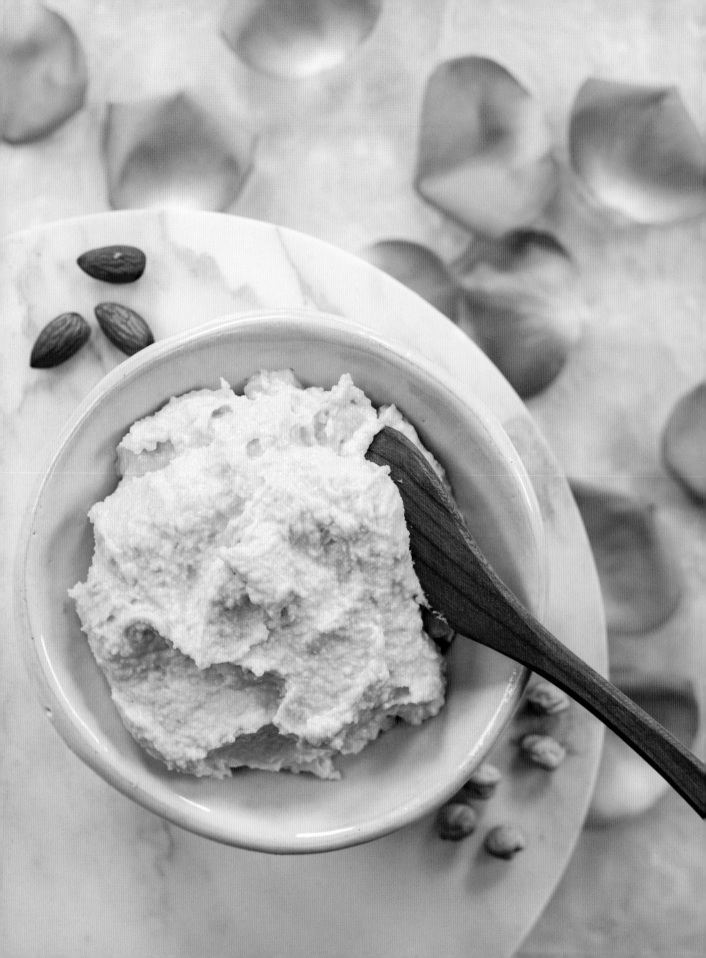

specialty recipe

ALMOND AND YOGURT BODY SCRUB

This recipe was inspired by the Ubtan, a traditional Ayurvedic beauty treatment. In India, Ubtans are made by combining a selection of medicinal herbs with crushed rose petals, almond meal, and chickpea flour. The mixture is then stirred into fresh yogurt and applied to the entire body as a mask before being massaged away. Sounds pretty luxurious, don't you think? My version is far more simple, but still combines the soothing and exfoliating richness of almond and yogurt. If you have it available, try adding a few drops of rose essential oil to this recipe for an especially indulgent experience.

INGREDIENTS

- ½ cup almond meal
- ½ cup chickpea flour
- ½ cup plain organic yogurt
- ¼ cup coconut milk, unsweetened or cow's milk
- ½ teaspoon rose or geranium essential oil (optional)

DIRECTIONS

Combine ingredients in a mixing bowl and stir well, adding additional yogurt if necessary.

HOW TO USE

I recommend starting this experience with a warm bath. After a good long soak your skin will be prime for pampering! Pat yourself dry, then start coating your arms, legs, and torso with the yogurt mixture. Relax for fifteen to twenty minutes to give the lactic acids in the yogurt time to loosen your dead skin cells. To avoid making a mess (or putting on a show for the rest of your household) I suggest lounging in an empty bath tub with a good book. If you prefer to be mobile, you can wrap your body in muslin or cheesecloth then throw on a bath robe that you won't mind dirtying up. When you are ready, massage the scrub in a slow circular motion until it crumbles away from your skin. Rinse your skin with warm water when you are finished scrubbing, using a little soap if you feel the need.

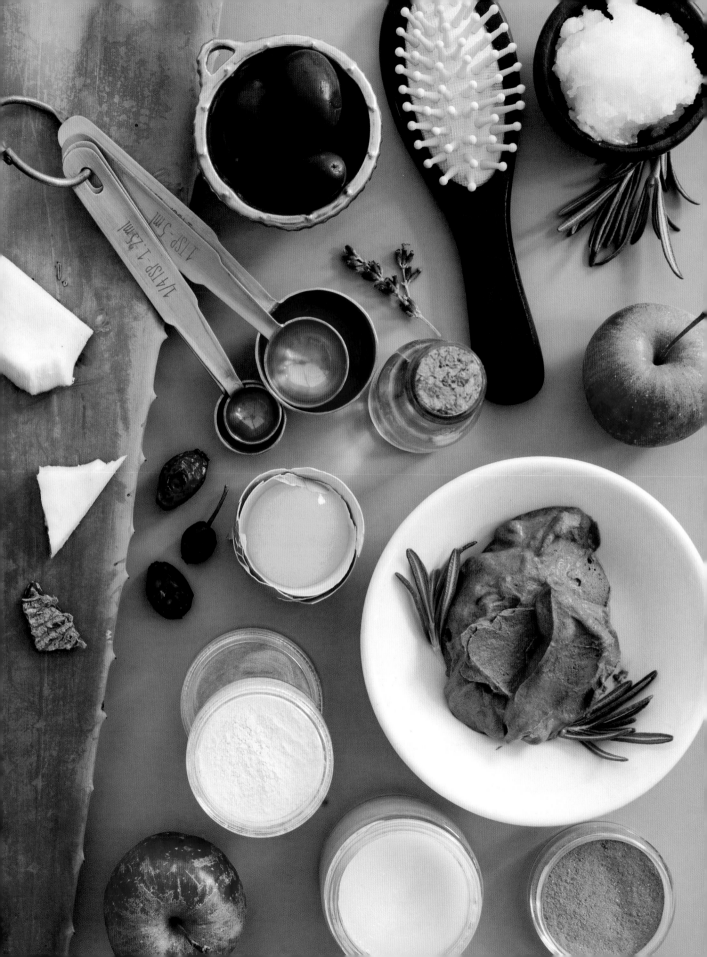

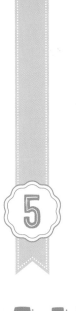

HAIR

Have you ever wondered why we shampoo? Did you know that shampoo wasn't introduced until the turn of the 20th century? In 1898, one of the world's first shampoos was invented in Germany. It wasn't until the 1930s that shampoo became popular in the United States. Before that time, hair washing was a monthly or bi-weekly event involving not much beyond soap and water. Our obsession with washing our hair on a daily basis has resulted in a sea of unbalanced scalps and frizzy heads—a far cry from the luxurious tresses commercial shampoos promise.

All in all, hair care is usually the most challenging aspect of a natural beauty routine, but it can also be the most rewarding. Commercial shampoos often include harsh detergents like SLS (sodium laurel sulfate) that strip the scalp of its natural oils. Conditioners use synthetic ingredients like silicone to give hair a silky and smooth appearance by coating the shafts. This can make your hair appear shiny and temporarily beautiful, but it does so at the cost of your hair's long-term health. By sealing your hair in additives like silicone, moisture is effectively » locked out, leading to hair that is dry, brittle, and easily broken.

The commercial shampoo and conditioner routine must be repeated constantly to keep up the cycle of strip, coat, and repeat. A natural routine works in a completely different way by encouraging your scalp to moisturize and protect your hair by restoring its natural balance. When given the chance, your scalp will produce just the right amount of sebum to keep your hair soft, smooth, and healthy. If necessary, your hair's moisture can be supplemented with natural oils, like avocado, virgin coconut, and watermelon seed. If you are feeling adventurous, you can even craft your own styling products like pomade, and texturizing scrunch spray.

A natural hair care routine usually results in hair that is less frizzy, better moisturized, and healthier. Some people even find their hair to grow stronger and faster after switching to a natural routine. Your hair may also show character that it hadn't previously. For example, after I settled into my all natural routine, I was pleasantly surprised to find curls, body, and highlights that I hadn't see in my hair since I was a teenager.

WHAT TO EXPECT

Unfortunately, resetting the balance of your scalp won't happen overnight. In fact, switching to a natural routine usually means suffering through a pretty intense adjustment period lasting between two

FAQ

What is the No-Poo Method?

No-Poo, as in *shampoo*, is a term used to describe any method of washing your hair that forgoes conventional shampoo. While the baking soda wash is probably the most famous no-poo recipe, there are countless other methods and techniques out there to experiment with. People everywhere are embracing natural and DIY hair care like never before. As the trend continues to draw people away from beauty shops and into their own kitchens I think of it less as a method and more as a movement. If you want to discover more no-poo method and recipes beyond what I've shared in this book I recommend checking out *thenopoomethod.com*, a site entirely dedicated to ditching shampoo!

to eight weeks. When cut off from the cycle of shampooing and conditioning, your scalp will go through phases of over and under producing sebum until it gets the balance just right. You can expect a lot of bad hair days during this adjustment period. You may also have to tweak your technique or recipes during this time, which adds another challenge to the mix.

This might all sound a little daunting, but once you get past the initial adjustment period the reward is a happier, healthier head of hair, and a simple routine that will continue to improve as time goes on. Once your routine is established, you may find that using natural products is actually quicker and easier than using conventional shampoos and conditioners. While you can rinse your hair as often as you like, you'll only need to wash your hair two or three times a week.

FOUR STEPS TO HEALTHIER HAIR

While switching to a natural routine is one of the best things you can do for your hair and scalp, products aren't the only opportunity for improvement. There are quite a few methods and techniques that can also help keep your hair healthy and beautiful.

- **Use a Bristle Brush.** Using a bristle brush, preferably made from natural fibers, can help distribute your scalp's natural oils throughout the length of your hair. Past generations would swear by brushing hair with one hundred strokes a day as the secret to keeping long, lustrous locks. Just make sure to clean your brush regularly so that harmful bacteria won't build up within it's bristles. Remove hair and debris from the brush using a small comb weekly. Every month or so you should also wash the brush with a gentle soap (like castile) and warm water.

- **Wash with Warm Water.** Washing or rinsing your hair in very hot water can strip the natural oils from your scalp, disrupting the balance that natural hair care relies on. It can also contribute to frizziness and breakage by forcing cuticles to open inappropriately on the hair shaft. Keep the water temperature mild to encourage healthy hair and scalp.

- **Dry with Care.** If you're in the habit of rubbing your hair with a towel to dry, you could be responsible for serious damage. Rough treatment of wet hair can cause breakage, frizz, and dullness. Instead of scrunching or rubbing your hair with a towel, gently squeeze or pat your hair. Serious hair gurus recommend investing in a special hair towel made just for pampering damp tresses. DIY hair aficionados recommend using an old t-shirt as jersey fabrics are more gentle than the terry cloth in towels. After removing excess water with a towel, blow dry it using a cool setting. Heat should only be increased for styling. Attaching a diffuser to your blow dryer can also be help cut down on frizz and damage.

- **Sleep on Silk.** If you are experiencing breakage or frizziness there may be some room for improvement in your bedroom. While we sleep, our hair rubs against sheets and pillowcases that are often made of fibers that aren't kind to hair (cotton, polyester, etc.). Stop those snags, snarls, and tangles by making sure that your head rests against a slippery fabric. Silk is perfect for this purpose. Silk pillowcases or head wraps are wonderful solutions.

everyday recipe

BAKING SODA WASH

A simple solution of water and baking soda is the cornerstone of the no-poo movement, and all it takes to keep excess oil and grime from building up on your scalp. Making the jump from conventional shampoo to a no-poo method is probably the biggest change you'll make when switching to a natural routine. There is a long period of adjustment involved in switching from shampoo to baking soda (around six to eight weeks) but if you can hang tough and take the time to troubleshoot as necessary, you'll be rewarded with a whole new head of hair that is healthy, gorgeous, and totally non-toxic.

This Baking Soda Wash can be used up to two to three times per week. It's important to rinse your hair well after using the Baking Soda Wash as any leftover residue can leave your hair feeling dry and tacky. Baking soda residue can also irritate your scalp by disrupting your skin's pH. Baking Soda Wash should always be followed with an Apple Cider Vinegar Rinse. The rinse will help remove leftover baking soda and balance the pH of your scalp. You may also need to use a dab of Conditioning Oil now and then to supplement moisture.

Be very, very gentle when massaging the wash into your scalp. Rubbing too hard can cause breakage, especially when you are just getting started with this method.

PERSONAL STORIES

Life After Shampoo

As I mixed up my first bottles of baking soda wash and vinegar rinse, I wondered for a moment if I'd finally gone off the deep end. Was I really giving up shampoo? I had my doubts, especially during the long transition period. One day I would wake up with greasy, knotty hair. Then the next day I would find it unexpectedly silky and light. By the time I reached the six week mark I had developed a serious love/hate relationship with the baking soda method. On one hand, my hair was shiny, smooth, and brimming with curls. At the same time it felt a little dry and crispy—no matter how many times I tried adjusting my recipes.

Finally, I tried smoothing a few drops of virgin coconut oil into my hair after washing it. That did the trick. Suddenly my hair felt as soft and pretty as it had on my best days using shampoo and conditioner. As the weeks I spent shampoo-free continued, my hair needed the coconut oil less and less. Now that I've been at it for two years, my hair has completely balanced out. I almost never have to add any oil or product to keep it looking shiny and smooth. I wash my hair about twice a week, rinsing it with plain water in between if I need to blow it out for styling.

Suffice to say the hate side of my relationship with no-poo is long gone. My hair hasn't been this healthy since I was a teenager. Not only is it glossy and full of body—its natural highlights have emerged, painting my head in a rainbow of colors that I thought had abandoned me in my thirties. It turns out that my hair hadn't pooped out with maturity. Its beauty had just been masked under a layer of silicone and sulfate.

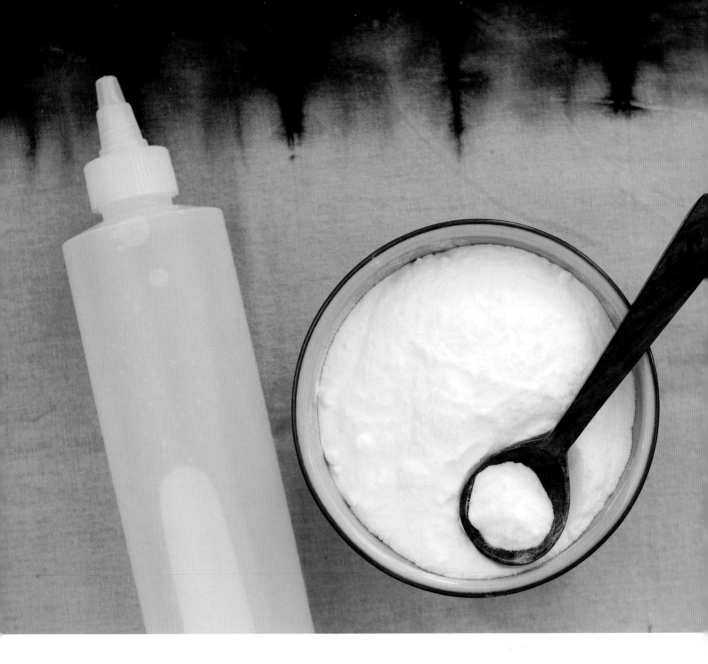

INGREDIENTS

- 1 teaspoon baking soda
- 1 cup water

DIRECTIONS

Combine ingredients in a plastic squirt bottle and shake well.

HOW TO USE

Squirt a liberal amount of the Baking Soda Wash into the scalp of your wet hair. You don't need to apply the wash directly to the ends of your hair. Gently massage your scalp for about thirty seconds (don't leave the baking soda on your hair for too long or it could cause irritation), then rinse thoroughly with water. Follow with the Apple Cider Vinegar Rinse.

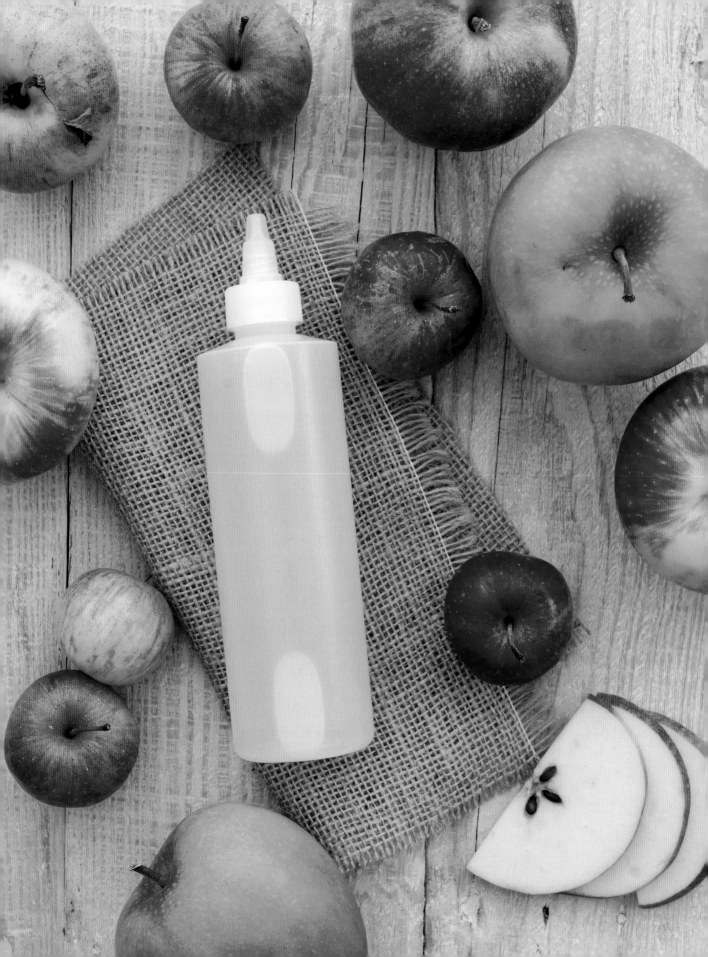

everyday recipe

APPLE CIDER VINEGAR RINSE

No matter how you plan on washing your hair, the Apple Cider Vinegar Rinse can be helpful as a conditioner. Apple Cider Vinegar helps keep your scalp healthy by balancing its pH, soothing dry, itchy skin, and discouraging dandruff. This rinse also works as a detangler, leaving your hair feeling soft, silky, and easy to manage. It's very important to use the Apple Cider Vinegar Rinse after any of the natural hair washes in this book—especially the Baking Soda Wash.

PROFESSIONAL HELP

Staying Natural at the Salon

I felt a little awkward the first time I went for a haircut after switching to an all-natural hair care routine. Asking my stylist not to use shampoo when she rinsed my hair left my cheeks blushing in embarrassment. What if she thought my hair was dirty? What if I gross her out or she thinks I'm a total weirdo? I almost chickened out and cheated on my no-poo method, but in the end I stayed strong and my stylist's reaction was pretty much zilch. She didn't care one bit that I didn't use shampoo!

After going through the scenario several times over the past few years I've found that most stylists don't bat an eye when I refuse shampoo and conditioner. I think this is partly due to the fact that hair care is such a personal thing. Forgoing shampoo and conditioner before a cut is probably not the strangest request a stylist hears. Another factor is the growing popularity of no-poo and other natural hair care methods. These days it's not all that odd to stop using shampoo. Since stylists are often in the know when it comes to the latest hair care trends, it's really not that surprising to find that they are hip to no-poo and natural hair care.

Since you'll be skipping the customary shampoo before your cut, I recommend making sure your hair is nice and clean before you show up to the salon.

I like to wash my hair one day before my appointment. It's a good idea to let your stylist know right away that you don't use shampoo and that you'd like to have your hair rinsed with plain water. If you run into a stylist who poo-poo's your no-poo ways, stay strong. You've worked hard to balance your scalp. While the occasional shampoo won't totally destroy your hair, it could spark another (probably shorter) adjustment period.

As for styling products used at the salon, the choice is up to you. When you are getting your hair done be sure to speak up, and let your stylist know if you have a preference regarding what he or she does or does not use. However, don't expect them to have natural alternatives on hand if you refuse their standard products. If you do decide to make an exception to your usual natural routine the repercussions can be hard to predict. Your hair and scalp might go through another short adjustment period. Then again, you may get through such a deviation with no drama at all.

Remember—it's your hair. You have every right to specify how it is cared for at the salon. Whether you are there to get a haircut, updo, or a blowout, make sure to call the shots with confidence.

Apple Cider Vinegar Rinse (continued)

› INGREDIENTS ‹

- ▫ 1 tablespoon apple cider vinegar
- ▫ 1 cup water

› DIRECTIONS ‹

Combine ingredients in a squeeze bottle
and shake.

› HOW TO USE ‹

After washing and rinsing your hair with water,
douse it liberally with vinegar rinse. Massage the
rinse into your hair and let it sit for at least one
minute. I like to leave the rinse on as I wash the
rest of my body, then soak my hair with water to
remove the vinegar rinse. Make sure you spend
enough time removing the vinegar rinse from
your hair. I usually spend at least a full minute or
two running water over my hair before leaving
the shower. This will keep your hair from smelling
like vinegar when it dries.

TROUBLESHOOTING ‹

Hair Smells Like Vinegar

There are a few factors that could be contributing
to a lingering vinegar scent on your hair. The first
thing to consider is how well you are rinsing out the
Apple Cider Vinegar Rinse. Try rinsing your hair with
water for twice as long as you usually do to see if
that helps. The next thing to do is double-check the
ratio of vinegar to water in the Apple Cider Vinegar
rinse and the ratio of baking soda to water in the
Baking Soda Wash (if you are using one). If either
solution is too strong it can leave residue, which
the vinegar scent can cling to. You can try reducing
the amount of vinegar or baking soda in your
solutions to see if that helps get rid of any lingering
scent. Finally, take a look at your water. Hard water
can make natural hair care a bit more challenging.
Check out the *Troubleshooting: Hard Water* section
on page 103 for more information.

ask a
NATURAL BEAUTY
EXPERT

Q: Do you have any tips for
keeping up with a natural
DIY routine?

A: Transitioning to natural beauty
care is truly a journey. Because everyone
is unique when it comes to body chemistry and
preferences, my suggestion is to embrace the
process and keep trying until you find something
that works. There is an element of perseverance that
is required when it comes to natural beauty care.

Andrea Fabry, it-takes-time.com

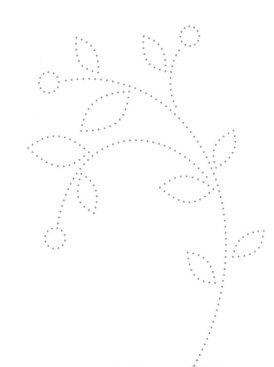

everyday recipe

ROSEMARY PALE ALE SHAMPOO BARS

If you aren't quite ready to give up shampoo—or if you've discovered that no-poo methods just don't work for you, you might want to consider a solid shampoo bar. Shampoo bars are soaps that have been specifically formulated for hair care. They offer the same kind of cleansing benefit of shampoo, but can be found or made in natural varieties that omit nasty ingredients like sulfates, parabens, and synthetic fragrance. Shampoo bars are also a good choice for people who simply must wash their hair on a daily basis. While your scalp would probably be happier if you cut down washes to two or three times per week, shampoo bars are gentle enough for daily use.

This particular recipe is a favorite of mine for hair care. It includes rich, moisturizing oils, detoxifying clay, and a splash of hoppy beer. Hops are excellent for adding softness and shine to hair, making them a natural match for shampoo bars. Like most natural hair cleansers, this shampoo should be followed with the Apple Cider Vinegar Rinse. Rhassoul clay is my preferred choice for this recipe, but if you don't have it handy, kaolin clay will do.

When purchasing soap base to work with, look for soaps made with pure saponified oils. Castile bars from Vermont Soap, Austin Natural Soap, or Castile rebatch base from Bramble Berry all work really well. Avoid any bars or bases that contain salt, as the soap won't melt as easily.

TROUBLESHOOTING

Hard Water

If you are experiencing dry frizzy hair, a lingering vinegar scent, or an itchy, irritated scalp, the hardness of your water could be the cause. If you've tried the other troubleshooting tips provided for these issues, it's time to take a look at your water. You can test your water for hardness with a kit from the hardware store, or by filling a clear plastic bottle halfway with water and a few drops of dish soap. Shake the bottle to form suds. The bottle should fill to the brim with big fluffy bubbles. If the suds don't form, that's a sign of hard water. The less suds there are, the harder your water may be.

Hard water contains a heavier load of minerals than usual. This can cause homemade hair washes to over cleanse, stripping too much oil from the hair and scalp. It can also prevent the Apple Cider Vinegar Rinse from removing residue effectively. There are ways to get around the problem hard water presents. One solution is to make your washes and rinse recipes using distilled water. This should help cut down on the effects the hard water has on your hair. Doing a second rinse with the Apple Cider Vinegar Rinse is another step you can take to work around hard water. If you'd rather solve the problem by eliminating your hard water, consider installing a filtering shower head or a water-softening system in your home.

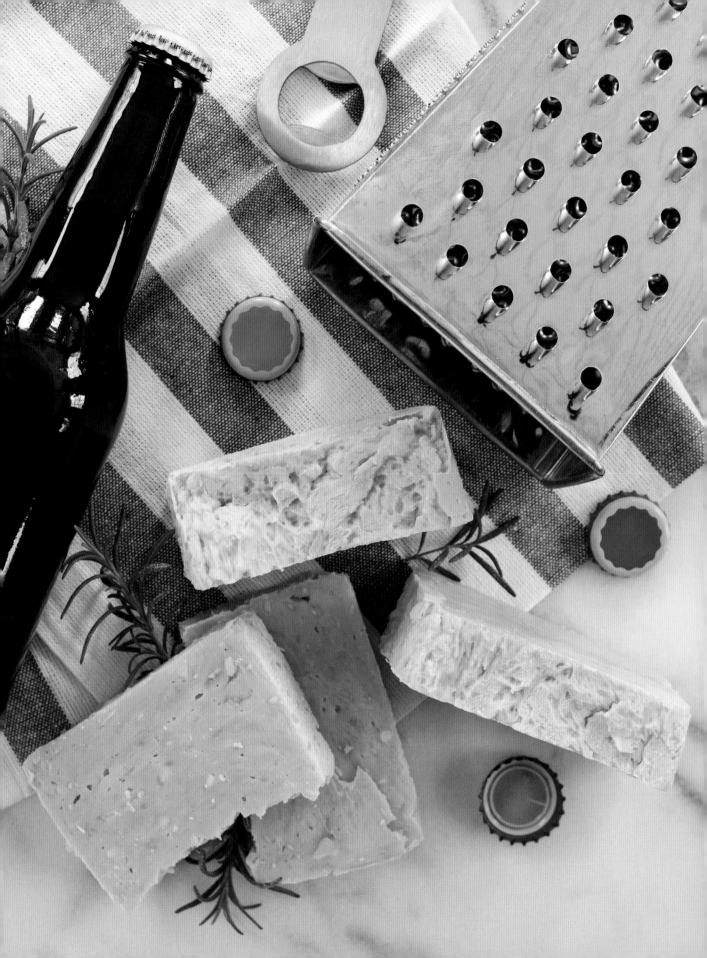

Rosemary Pale Ale Shampoo Bars (continued)

> INGREDIENTS <

- 1 pound natural castile bar soap, shredded
- ½ cup and 2 tablespoons pale ale (or any type of strong, hoppy beer)
- 2 tablespoons rhassoul or kaolin clay
- 1 tablespoon jojoba oil
- 1 tablespoon avocado oil
- 2 teaspoons rosemary essential oil

> DIRECTIONS <

Combine the shredded soap and ½ cup pale ale in a double boiler or crock pot set to low. Heat the mixture, stirring often, until fully melted. In a separate bowl, combine the remaining 2 tablespoons of pale ale with the clay. Add the clay mixture, jojoba oil, and avocado oil to the soap pot and stir well. Transfer to a silicone mold or a wooden mold lined with wax paper. Allow the soap to cool and set until it is hard enough to handle. This could take up to three days. When the soap has hardened, gently remove it from the mold and slice it into four bars. Set the bars on a rack to dry for an additional one to three weeks. The bars are ready to use when they are fully hardened and dry. For photos of this process, check out page 18.

> HOW TO USE <

Wet your hair, then work the bar into a rich lather between your palms. Apply the lather to your head, then gently massage it directly into your scalp. You don't need to apply the shampoo to the ends of your hair. Rinse well, then follow with the Apple Cider Vinegar Rinse.

TROUBLESHOOTING

Hair is Too Greasy or Tacky

There are few fixes you can try if your hair is feeling consistently greasy after the adjustment period has ended. First try applying the Apple Cider Vinegar rinse an additional time after every wash. This will give the vinegar a second chance to clarify your hair. Next, take a look at your washing method. If you are using the Baking Soda Wash, try reducing the amount of baking soda in your recipe by half. If you are using a shampoo bar, try making a batch of Rosemary Pale Ale Shampoo Bars without the added jojoba or avocado oils. No matter which washing method you use, you may want to try leaving the Vinegar Rinse on for an additional minute or two or washing your hair a little more often. Everyone is different, so you'll need to find the frequency of washing that works best for you.

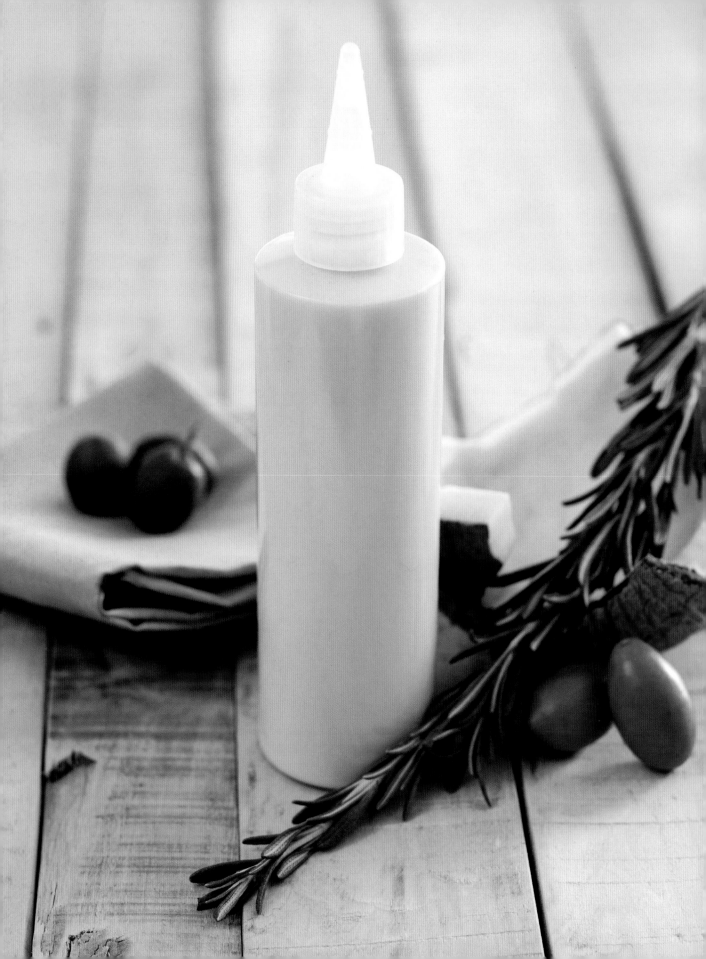

everyday recipe

COCONUT MILK WASH

The coconut is a wondrous thing. How the same amazing fruit offers the benefits of cleansing, conditioning, and even astringency is pretty amazing. This hair wash recipe is a great solution for anyone who wants a simple alternative to the baking soda method or has found other methods to be drying or irritating. The Coconut Milk Wash has a closer pH to your scalp than the Baking Soda Wash and combines soothing aloe vera gel with the healing powers of coconut.

Be sure to use coconut milk specifically for this recipe. Other coconut ingredients, like coconut water, coconut juice, or coconut cream won't work as well in this formula.

INGREDIENTS

- ¼ cup coconut milk, unsweetened
- ⅓ cup liquid castile soap
- ½ teaspoon jojoba oil
- ½ teaspoon avocado oil
- 15 drops rosemary essential oil (optional)
- 15 drops peppermint essential oil (optional)

DIRECTIONS

Combine ingredients in a squeeze bottle and shake well.

HOW TO USE

Shake the bottle well before each use. Wet your hair and squirt one to three teaspoons of the mixture onto your scalp. Massage the mixture gently into your scalp, building up a rich lather. Rinse well and follow with the Apple Cider Vinegar Rinse. This mixture will last at room temperature for a few days, but should be refrigerated for any longer periods. It's helpful to store the full batch in the fridge while keeping a smaller portion in the shower. Refrigerated, it will stay fresh for up to two weeks.

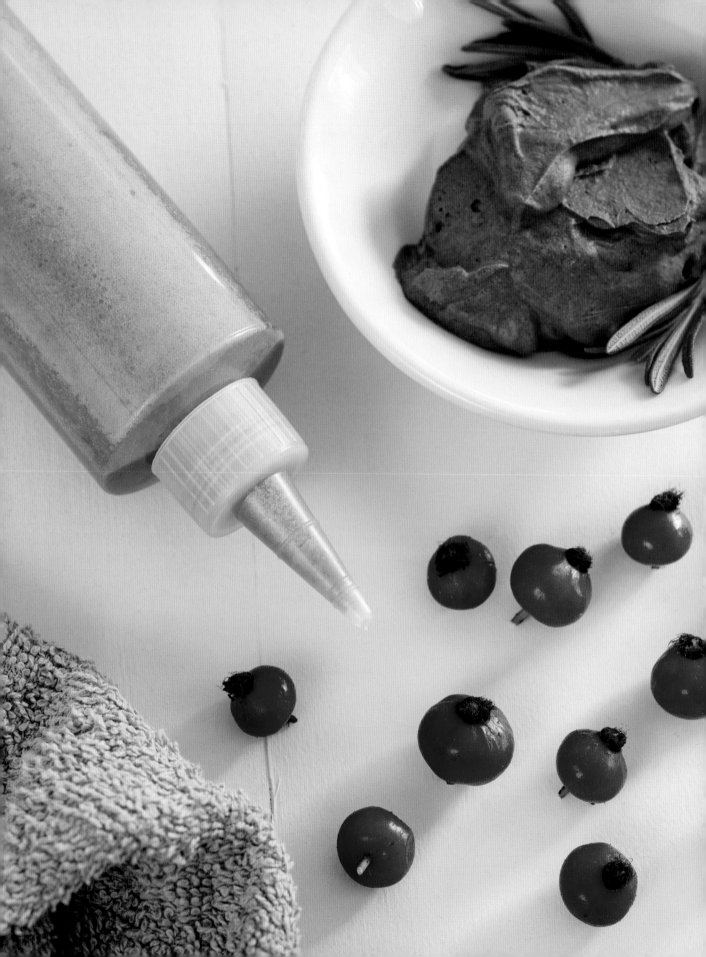

everyday recipe

RHASSOUL CLAY HAIR WASH

Washing your hair with clay might seem just about as wacky as washing your face with oil. Though it does sound a little counterintuitive, clay washing has actually been around for a very long time. In fact, the word *rhassoul* comes from an Arabic word meaning *to wash*. This clay wash recipe uses deep-cleaning rhassoul clay to remove dirt, grime, and excess oils from the scalp. If you have dry hair, add ½ teaspoon jojoba oil to the recipe to add back a little moisture. Peppermint essential oil can be added to give the recipe an energizing lift. Or rosemary essential oil can be used to help balance the scalp and increase shine.

INGREDIENTS

- ½ cup water
- 1 tablespoon rhassoul clay
- ½ teaspoon rose hip seed oil (optional)
- ⅛ teaspoon peppermint essential oil or rosemary essential oil (optional)

DIRECTIONS

Combine the water and clay in a small mixing bowl and stir to combine. Transfer the mixture to a squirt bottle, then add the jojoba oil and peppermint essential oil, if using. Shake well to combine the ingredients.

HOW TO USE

Wet your hair thoroughly, shake the bottle vigorously, then apply a generous amount of clay wash to the roots of your hair. It helps to work in sections to make sure you cover your entire head. Gently massage the mixture into your scalp being careful not to break your hair by scrubbing too hard. When you've coated your whole head, let it sit for about two minutes before rinsing it out with warm water. Follow with the Apple Cider Vinegar Rinse. This recipe makes enough wash for one or two sessions, depending on the length and thickness of your hair. Any leftovers can be stored in the refrigerator for up to one week.

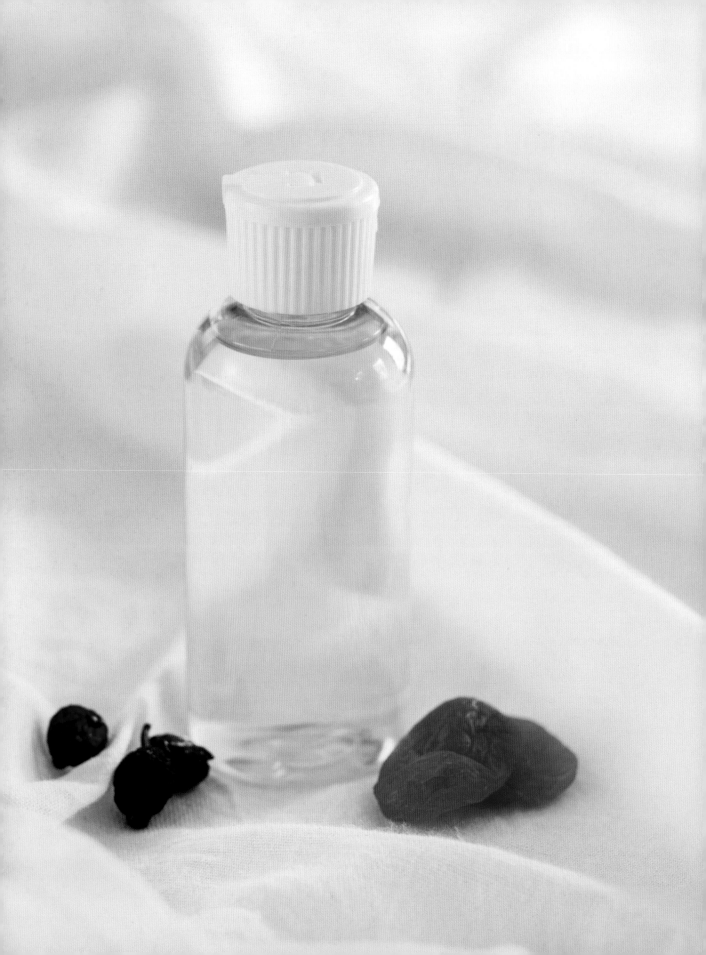

everyday recipe
CONDITIONING OIL BLEND

After switching to a natural hair care routine your hair may be a little dry now and then. This happens most in the first months of your new routine. While your scalp is learning to produce the right amount of oil to keep your hair moisturized it may be necessary to supplement that moisture with oil. Any of the carrier oils used in this recipe could be used alone to moisturize the hair, but together they create a well-balanced blend that suits most hair types very well. Virgin coconut oil adds light moisture—perfect for hair that tends toward oiliness. Apricot kernel, watermelon seed, or rose hip seed oil add a medium amount of moisture. Avocado oil and jojoba oil should be used only on very dry hair.

This recipe combines these oils, making a blend that works nicely for most hair. Conditioning oils are potent, so most people need only a few drops to moisturize their entire head of hair. Determining the amount to use takes a trial and error. Pay attention to how your hair reacts to the amount of oil in the recipe and use fewer or more drops in the future, as needed. In general, thick or curly hair can handle more oil than thin or straight hair..

I prefer to apply hair oil when my hair is damp—preferably following my usual wash and rinse routine. This helps distribute the oil further, avoiding a greasy, heavy feel. You may find that your hair absorbs oil really well—in which case you could probably get away with adding Conditioning Oil to dry hair.

> INGREDIENTS <

- 2 ounces virgin coconut oil
- 1 ounce watermelon seed oil or apricot kernel oil
- ½ ounce rose hip seed oil
- ½ ounce jojoba oil

> DIRECTIONS <

Warm the coconut oil in a double boiler or crockpot set to low until fully melted. Remove the oil from the heat, then add the other oils. Stir well, then transfer the oil blend to a 4-ounce bottle.

> HOW TO USE <

Start by using a dropper to place the oil in the palm of your hand. If you have short hair, use 2 to 4 drops. Use 4 to 8 for medium length hair, and 8 to 15 for long hair. Rub the oil between your palms, then rub the ends of your hair between your palms, working the oil into the tips of the strands. Rub any excess oil into the midsection of your hair next. You won't need to apply the oil to the roots of your hair, as that area will be moisturized by your scalp.

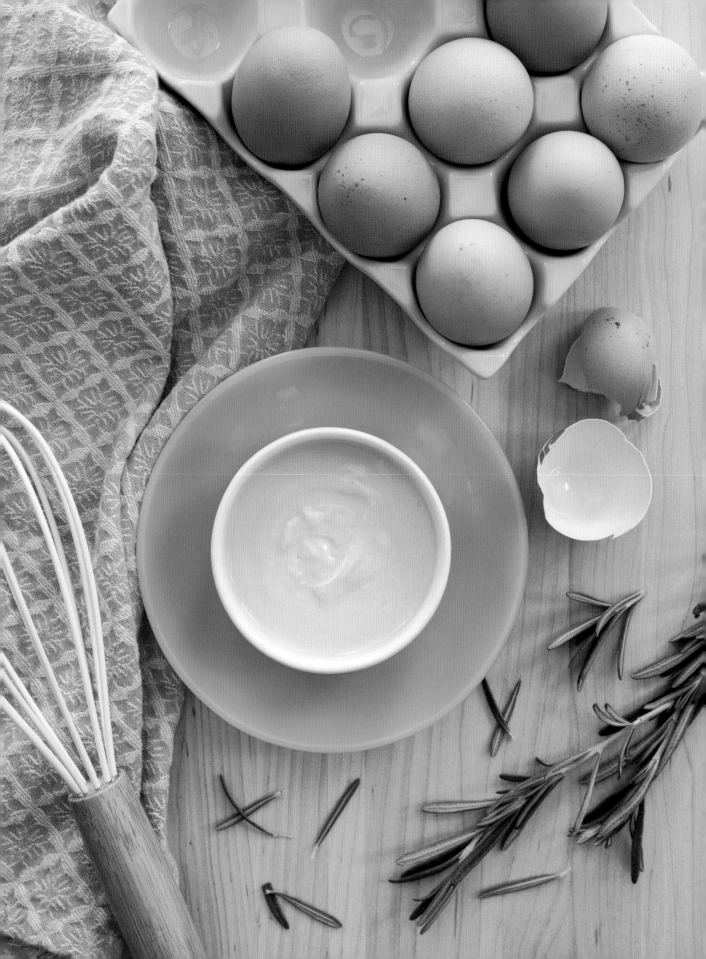

specialty recipe
EGG YOLK HAIR MASQUE

Mayonnaise is a classic ingredient for DIY beauty, used long before natural beauty became trendy. This homemade hair treatment became popular back when beauty queens bathed in buttermilk, and a gal could ditch a night out by using the excuse of staying home to wash her hair. While not every home remedy has a foot in scientific validity, this particular method of hair conditioner has a lot going for it. The cholesterol in eggs can help strengthen hair, making it less likely to break and dry out. Another main ingredient in mayo is vinegar—which balances pH and encourages softness. The final main ingredient in mayonnaise is vegetable oil—something we know can act as a deep conditioner.

This recipe takes the virtues of mayonnaise a step further by including apple cider vinegar and a blend of coconut, jojoba, avocado, and rose hip seed oils. A few drops of rosemary essential oil finishes this recipe off with a little scalp balancing action. Hair masques, like this one, provide deep-conditioning, so you don't want to use them every day. Depending on how thirsty your hair is, you can use this masque once a week, every other week, once a month, or whenever the mood strikes you.

This recipe calls for a pasteurized egg to reduce the chances of contaminating your shower (or your body) with salmonella. Many grocery stores now carry pasteurized eggs (sometimes called safe eggs), but if you can't find them, this recipe can be sterilized by heating in a double boiler until it comes to 165 degrees. The texture will change quite a bit, but it should still provide great benefits to your hair.

TROUBLESHOOTING

Hair is Too Dry or Frizzy

It may be possible that you are washing your hair too often. It's important to give your scalp time to replace the natural oils that keep it healthy between washes. Try washing a little less frequently, and if that doesn't help right away, consider supplementing your scalp's moisture with a healthy oil. You can use the Conditioning Oil recipe in this book, or go for something more simple, like rubbing a few drops of plain organic virgin coconut oil or rose hip seed oil into the ends of your hair. Doing an occasional deep conditioning treatment, like the Egg Yolk Hair Masque, can also help improve your hair's overall moisture. Another thing that can cause your hair to be dry or frizzy is hard water. Check out the section titled *Troubleshooting: Hard Water* for tips on how to battle hard water.

Egg Yolk Hair Masque (continued)

INGREDIENTS

- ▢ 1 pasteurized egg yolk*
- ▢ 3 teaspoons apple cider vinegar
- ▢ ¼ cup virgin coconut oil, melted
- ▢ ¼ cup jojoba oil
- ▢ ¼ cup avocado oil
- ▢ ¼ rose hip seed oil
- ▢ ¼ teaspoon rosemary essential oil

DIRECTIONS

Combine the egg yolk and vinegar in a small mixing bowl, then whisk together. In a second bowl, stir together the coconut, jojoba, avocado, and rose hip seed oils with the rosemary essential oil. Begin whisking the egg mixture and slowly pour a few drops of the oil mixture into it. Whisk it for a few seconds to get the emulsion started, then slowly drizzle the rest of the oil into the bowl as you whisk continuously. Continue whisking until all of the oil has been added. The mixture should thicken and turn opaque as the oils and vinegar emulsify.

* See page 113 for directions on how to make this recipe with an unpasturized egg yolk.

HOW TO USE

Apply the fresh masque mixture to your damp hair, making sure to start at the scalp. Massage the mixture into your scalp gently, then slowly work it down to the ends. Moisten a medium-sized towel with hot water, then wring it out so that it is damp, but not dripping wet. Pin or tie back your hair, then cover it with the hot towel. Let the masque sit in your hair for twenty to thirty minutes before rinsing it out. Follow with your usual cleanser and the Apple Cider Vinegar Rinse.

This masque is best used when fresh, but if necessary you can refrigerate any leftover portion for up to one week.

specialty recipe

NATURAL DETANGLER

Marshmallow root makes a super slippery tea when steeped in boiling water. This special herb can be found online at certain soap making and herb suppliers and sometimes in the natural tea section of grocery stores. Since this detangler is left in the hair to dry, I like to add a pleasant smelling hydrosol such as rose, neroli, or lavender to the mix. If you are prone to dandruff or have an itchy scalp, try using rosemary hydrosol instead. If you don't have hydrosol on hand, substitute that portion of the recipe with extra water.

INGREDIENTS

- 2 tablespoons marshmallow root powder
- 1 cup water
- 1 cup hydrosol (neroli, rose, lavender, or rosemary)

DIRECTIONS

Bring water to a boil, then add the marshmallow root. Turn off the heat and let the root steep in the water for thirty minutes. Strain the mixture into a 16-ounce bottle and discard the solids. Add the hydrosol, then shake well.

HOW TO USE

The detangler should be packaged in a spray bottle to make application easy. Spritz the detangler on to damp or dry hair before combing. The detangler will last about two weeks in the refrigerator and can be used cold or at room temperature.

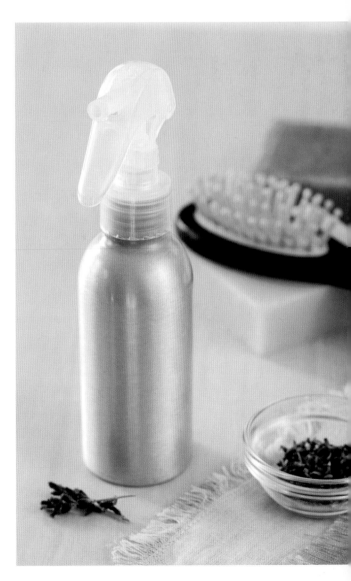

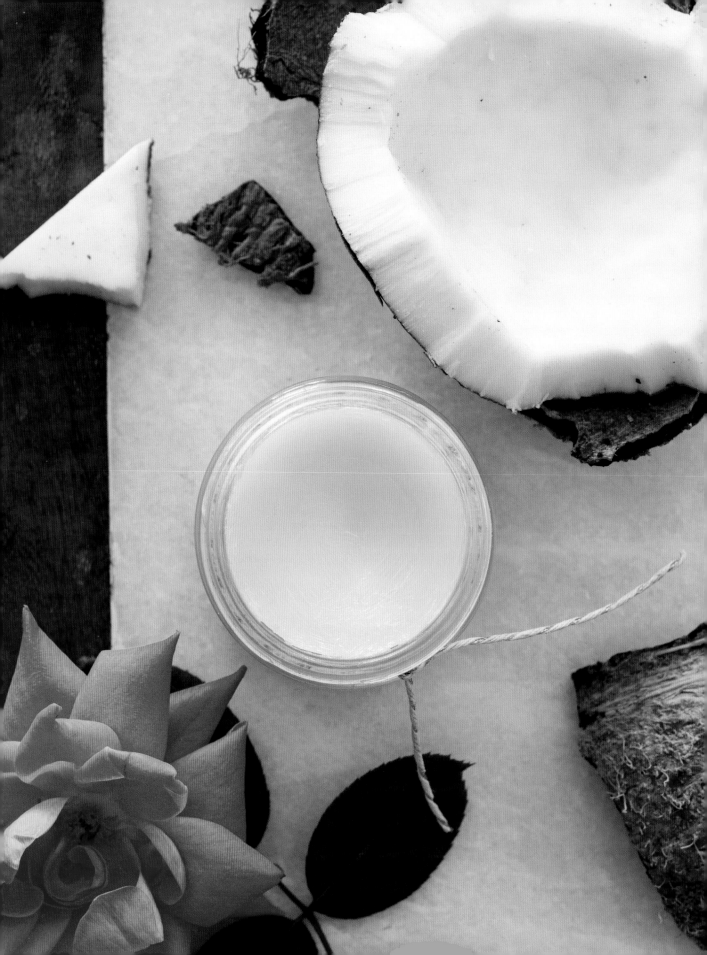

specialty recipe

POMADE

This soft, waxy balm can help add texture to your hair while boosting it with conditioning oils. Use pomade to spike, twist, or style your hair to your heart's content without worrying about toxic ingredients like polymers and fragrance. A touch of neroli or rose essential oil can be added to give the product a pretty scent.

INGREDIENTS

- 2 tablespoons virgin coconut oil
- 1 tablespoon apricot kernel oil
- 1 tablespoon jojoba oil
- 2 tablespoons beeswax pellets
- ¼ teaspoon neroli or rose essential oil (optional)

DIRECTIONS

Combine the coconut oil, apricot oil, jojoba oil, and beeswax in a double boiler and heat until the ingredients are fully melted. Remove the mixture from the heat, wait a few moments, before adding the essential oil (if using). Stir well, then carefully pour the melted balm into a 4-ounce jar. Allow the balm to cool and harden completely before use.

HOW TO USE

Scoop a small dab of pomade into the palm of your hand, then rub your hands together to soften it up. Rub the mixture into your hair wherever you'd like to add a little extra weight, hold, or texture.

PROFESSIONAL HELP

Coloring Hair

There aren't too many 100% natural options out there for coloring your hair. When it comes to lightening, a few squirts of lemon juice and a day in the sun will certainly lift it a shade or two, but the results are unpredictable. Herbal recipes using ingredients like henna, black walnut powder, and sage can be used to tint your hair. These recipes can actually provide some very lovely results, but you can't expect the kind of intense color that you would find with a trip to the salon or even a box of at-home hair color.

Commercial dyes often use toxic ingredients to bleach and dye your hair. According to some studies, substances like resorcinol, ethanolamine, and parabens may cause endocrine disruption, organ toxicity, and serious skin irritation. Luckily, as awareness regarding cosmetic toxicity grows, safer options for professional hair color are becoming available. If you decide to make an exception to your natural beauty routine for the sake of professional color, look for salons that offer dyes without toxic ingredients like ammonia, resorcinol, ethanolamine, and parabens.

As for caring for color-treated hair, most natural hair care methods shouldn't cause hair color to fade, but they don't contain any special additives to make it last longer like you might find in commercial shampoos and conditioners.

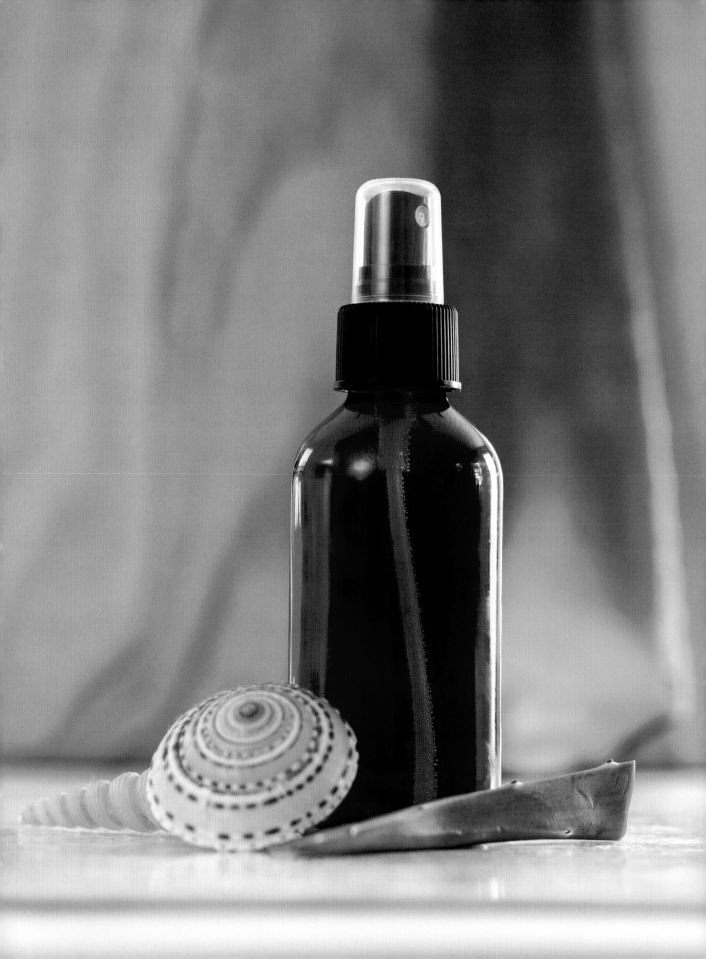

specialty recipe
SCRUNCH SPRAY

Sea salt is great for encouraging your hair's natural wave, curl, and texture to come out and play. By combining salt water with moisturizing aloe gel and the fruity floral scent of neroli hydrosol, you can capture the flirty spirit of beach hair without having to jump in the ocean!

INGREDIENTS

- 1 tablespoon sea salt
- ¼ cup water
- 2 tablespoons aloe vera gel
- 2 tablespoons neroli hydrosol

DIRECTIONS

Heat the water to a boil, then remove from heat. Stir in the salt, then allow the mixture to cool to room temperature. Combine the cooled salt water with the aloe vera gel and neroli hydrosol in a 4-ounce spray bottle, then shake well.

HOW TO USE

Package your Scrunch Spray in a spray bottle for easy application. Spritz the spray onto damp hair, then scrunch it in your palm as you blow dry or air dry your hair. The Scrunch Spray will last about two weeks in the refrigerator and can be used cold or at room temperature.

Natural Beauty Tip:
Use Hydrosols to Add Scent

Even though natural hair care has plenty of virtues, giving up the fun flirty scents of commercial shampoos and conditioners can be hard. We've grown accustomed to equating clean hair with sweet scents like coconut, apple, and flowers. It would be great if we could all just embrace the natural human aromas of our freshly cleaned heads, but it can be awfully hard to let go of our candy-scented cosmetics. Hydrosols offer a totally natural way to add safe aroma to your hair on an everyday basis. Just package your favorite hydrosol in a spray bottle and spritz it directly into your hair to add a splash of aroma. My personal favorite variety of hydrosol for this purpose is neroli, but you might prefer rose, lavender, lemon balm, or geranium.

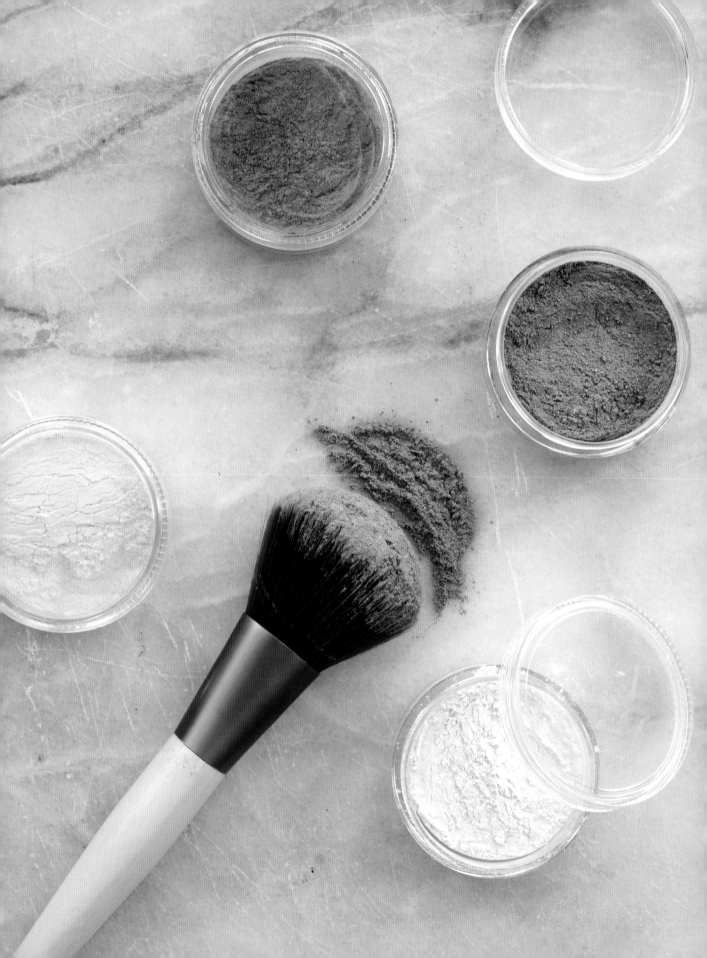

specialty recipe

DRY SHAMPOO

Using dry shampoo is a great way to tide your scalp over in between washes, or to take greasiness down a notch. Unlike most shampoos, dry shampoo doesn't actually clean your hair. Instead it keeps hair tidy in between washes by absorbing excess oils on your scalp. This simple hair powder is especially useful during the challenging weeks of the adjustment period between conventional and natural hair care methods. The powder is applied using a large cosmetic brush, dusting on just enough to absorb excess oil, giving your hair a temporary reprieve from the grips of the dreaded bad hair day. Cornstarch and kaolin are all that is needed to create a basic dry shampoo that is suitable for light-colored hair. If you have dark hair, try adding cocoa powder to make the powder less visible.

INGREDIENTS

- 1 tablespoon cornstarch
- 1 tablespoon kaolin clay
- 2 tablespoons cocoa powder
  (for use in dark hair only)

DIRECTIONS

Stir the cornstarch, kaolin clay, and cocoa powder (if using) together and transfer to a small jar, preferably one with a sifter.

HOW TO USE

Tap out a small shake of powder into a little dish. Swirl a large cosmetic brush into the powder then gently dust the roots of your hair with a light coating. Use your fingers to work the powder into your hair, smoothing away any visible patches.

TROUBLESHOOTING

Bad Hair Days

As much as I love natural hair care, I would be a liar if I told you that the whole thing was rainbows and sunshine. When you are getting ready to start things off, it's important to mentally prepare yourself for the rigors of the adjustment period. There will be some dark days ahead—days where your hair is greasy, grimy, frizzy, limp, dull, and sometimes downright devious. It helps to have a plan in place to tackle bad hair days. My best lines of defense were headbands, ponytails, and buns. Another thing that can assist in getting you through those days is dry shampoo. However you choose to defend against bad hair days, just hang in there. The longer you keep up your natural routine, the better your results will be, especially if you take the time to troubleshoot and make adjustments along the way.

APPENDIX

RESOURCES

Recipes, Tutorials, and Information on DIY Skin Care, Hair Care, and Soap Making

AromaWeb

A veritable essential oil encyclopedia, Aroma Web offers over one hundred essential oil profiles with benefits, safety, and usage information on each ingredient.
aromaweb.com

Artifact Girl

A site featuring beautiful natural skin care recipes from Narae Kim of Artifact Girl Cosmetics, a unique line of natural facial masques that focus on cultural traditions in skincare that are naturally natural.
artifactgirl.com

Blah Blah Magazine

Natural recipes and projects for beauty, home, and family from Cybele Masterman, a beauty therapist, makeup artist, journalist (and soon to be cosmetic chemist).
blahblahmagazine.com.au

Blythe Natural Living

Blythe shares her quick and easy plant based recipes (no soy, gluten, or dairy), her DIY therapeutic home spa treatments and all things natural lifestyle.
blythenaturalliving.com

Crunchy Betty

One of the best resources online for DIY natural beauty. Crunchy Betty features recipes, a lively community, and even a shop selling products and ingredients.
crunchybetty.com

It Takes Time

DIY projects and recipes for natural living from Andrea Fabry.
it-takes-time.com

Mary Makes Good

The author's personal blog features DIY beauty tutorials as well as recipes and projects for the home, kitchen, and family.
marymakesgood.com

The National Association for Holistic Aromonatherapy

NAHA publishes important safety information and further reading on the use of essential oils.
naha.org

Natural Beauty Workshop

A natural beauty blog owned by the cosmetic ingredient supplier, From Nature With Love. This site features hundreds of free recipes, detailed ingredient information, and more. Written by the author.
naturalbeautyworkshop.com

The Natural Solution Facebook Group

A forum for discussions on natural ingredients, methods, and techniques for cooking, beauty, home care, and more.
facebook.com/groups/NaturalSolution

The No Poo Method

An entire site dedicated to natural shampoo alternatives. The No Poo Method offers articles, links, and recipes to help you delve deeper into the world beyond shampoo.
thenopoomethod.com

Teach Soap

If you are interested in learning more about making your own soap, Teach Soap is an excellent place to get started. You can find recipes, tutorials, and a community forum to help get you started.
teachsoap.com

Supplies for DIY Skin Care, Hair Care, and Soap Making

Austin Natural Soap
All natural cold processed bar soaps.
austinsoap.com

Bramble Berry
Soap making ingredients including oils, butters, and rebatch base.
brambleberry.com

From Nature With Love
Wholesale supplier of 1,750+ natural and complementary ingredients used in skin care, hair care, and soap making. This is a great source for oils, butters, essential oils, hydrosols, exfoliants, clays, and packaging.
fromnaturewithlove.com

The Herb Bar
A great source for herbal ingredients and finished handmade products in Austin, Texas.
theherbbar.com

Mary Makes Good
Natural ingredients, DIY beauty kits, and finished natural products from the author.
marymakesgood.bigcartel.com

Mountain Rose Herbs
Another good resource for basic ingredients as well as finished natural products.
mountainroseherbs.com

Vermont Soap
All natural cold processed bar and liquid castile soaps.
vermontsoap.com

Further Reading on Ingredient Toxicity in Cosmetics

Campaign for Safe Cosmetics
Learn more about dangerous additives and ingredients used in cosmetics and how you can help join the fight to ban harmful substances from personal care products.
safecosmetics.org

Environmental Working Group
A leading resource for information on product safety, EWG's site features tools and articles to help you shop more safely for home and personal care products. The site also includes links to research and articles on why certain ingredients are considered unsafe.
ewg.org

EWG's Skin Deep Cosmetics Database
The Environmental Working Group has done an amazing job of compiling scientific data on almost any ingredient you might find in commercial home and personal care products. You can search Skin Deep's website or smart phone app by ingredient or by product to view ingredient information and safety ratings.
ewg.org/skindeep

Organic Consumer's Association
A great resource for learning more about the personal and ecological safety of consumer products. The Organic Consumer's Association focuses on campaigning for safer, more sustainable food, cosmetics, and consumer goods.
organicconsumers.org

Worksheet:

NATURAL BEAUTY RESULTS

NATURAL BEAUTY PRODUCT	INGREDIENTS

Copies of this worksheet available at *springhousepress.com*.

	OBSERVATIONS				
	1 DAY	3 DAYS	1 WEEK	2 WEEKS	1 MONTH

Worksheet:
MY BATHROOM CABINET CLEANSE

COMMERCIAL PRODUCT	NATURAL REPLACEMENT	DONE
		☐
		☐
		☐
		☐
		☐
		☐
		☐
		☐
		☐
		☐
		☐
		☐
		☐
		☐
		☐
		☐

Copies of this worksheet available at *springhousepress.com*.

INDEX

Index (continued)

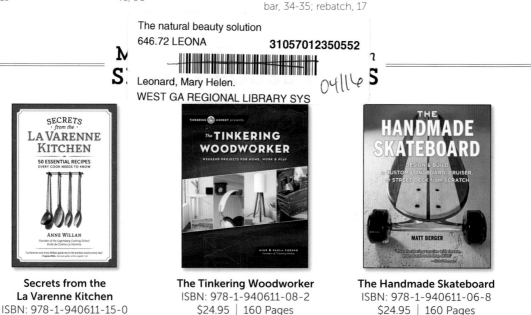

Secrets from the La Varenne Kitchen
ISBN: 978-1-940611-15-0
$17.95 | 136 Pages

The Tinkering Woodworker
ISBN: 978-1-940611-08-2
$24.95 | 160 Pages

The Handmade Skateboard
ISBN: 978-1-940611-06-8
$24.95 | 160 Pages

Look for these Spring House Press titles at your favorite bookstore or woodworking retailer. For more information or to order direct, visit *www.springhousepress.com* or call 717-208-3739.